Epidemiology of Healthcare-associated Infections in Australia

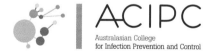

ACIPC
Australasian College
for Infection Prevention and Control

**Endorsed by the Australasian College
for Infection Prevention and Control (ACIPC)**
ACIPC is the peak body for infection prevention and
control professionals in the Australasian region.

This publication has been externally peer reviewed.

Epidemiology of Healthcare-associated Infections in Australia

RAMON Z. SHABAN

BSc(Med), BN, GradCertInfCon, PGDipPH&TM, MEd, MCommHealthPrac(Hons), PhD, RN, CICP-E, FCENA, FACN, FACIPC

Clinical Chair of Infection Prevention and Disease Control, Marie Bashir Institute for Infectious Diseases and Biosecurity and Susan Wakil School of Nursing and Midwifery, Faculty of Medicine and Health, University of Sydney, Camperdown, NSW, Australia

Associate Director (Engagement and Research), New South Wales Biocontainment Centre and the Department of Infection Prevention and Control, Division of Infectious Diseases and Sexual Health, Westmead Hospital and Western Sydney Local Health District, NSW, Australia

Senior Editor, Infection, Disease and Health

BRETT G. MITCHELL

PhD, MAdvPrac, DTN, CHealthM, BN, RN, CICP-E, FACIPC, FACN

Professor of Nursing, University of Newcastle, NSW, Australia

Conjoint Scholar, Central Coast Local Health District, NSW, Australia

Editor-in-Chief, Infection, Disease and Health

PHILIP L. RUSSO

PhD, MClinEpid, BN, RN, CICP-E, FACIPC, MACN

Associate Professor, Monash University, Victoria, Australia

Cabrini Health, Victoria, Australia

DEBOROUGH MACBETH

RN, PhD, CICP-E

Queensland, Australia

ELSEVIER

ELSEVIER

Elsevier Australia. ACN 001 002 357
(a division of Reed International Books Australia Pty Ltd)
Tower 1, 475 Victoria Avenue, Chatswood, NSW 2067

ISBN: 978-0-7295-4363-7

National Library of Australia Cataloguing-in-Publication Data

A catalogue record for this book is available from the National Library of Australia

Senior Content Strategist: Libby Houston
Content Project Manager: Sukanthi Sukumar
Edited by Leanne Peters
Proofread by Tim Learner
Cover Designer: Georgette Hall
Typeset by New Best-set Typesetters Ltd

Last digit is the print number: 9 8 7 6 5 4 3 2 1

CONTENTS

 View a video summary of the content

Foreword

Epidemiology of Healthcare-associated Infections in Australia (1st edition) is a new and important resource to help us better manage and prevent common but serious and often life-threatening complications of healthcare, namely healthcare-associated infections.

For the first time, this title brings together the publicly available data from three disparate sources—jurisdictional surveillance data, published peer-reviewed literature and hospital-acquired complication (HAC) healthcare-associated infection data—in an attempt to describe the burden of healthcare-associated infections in Australia. It looks critically at the importance of documenting the epidemiology of healthcare-associated infections in Australia and delves into the currently available data, providing the first comprehensive picture of the issue.

Epidemiology of Healthcare-associated Infections in Australia (1st edition) illustrates clearly the problems that arise from currently having three sets of data, each providing different answers about the burden of these common infections within Australia and within and between various states and territories. Australian states and territories are responsible for, and administer, their own systems. And as this title demonstrates, there are major problems with the utility of these data in light of the fact as there is no single unified national healthcare-associated infection surveillance system.

The authors do show that despite its flaws, some of the publicly available data give a very good insight into what is happening with infections, including *Staphylococcus aureus* blood stream infections and surgical site infections. However, it's only once we have more accurate, up-to-date, consistently defined and publicly available data that we can move to further improve infection prevention and control practices. Accurate and timely information assists in evaluating jurisdictional and national initiatives to reduce healthcare-associated infections, as well as learn from successes and identify areas of concern in a timely manner. This is particularly relevant for urinary tract infections with the increasing numbers associated with high-risk procedures, such as the use of indwelling urinary catheters and increasing antimicrobial resistance.

Epidemiology of Healthcare-associated Infections in Australia (1st edition) highlights the importance of and need for a national system for collecting data systemically and accurately, and making it publicly available in a timely fashion. This is vital if we want to make better progress towards decreasing the numbers of these infections and preventing them from occurring to begin with.

Authors Professor Ramon Shaban, Professor Brett Mitchell, Associate Professor Philip Russo and Dr Deborough Macbeth bring extensive individual and collective expertise and practical experience as on-the-ground infection control practitioners in preparing this critically important contribution that will help us all to prevent and control healthcare-associated infections in Australia.

Professor Peter Collignon AM
Patron, Australasian College for Infection Prevention and Control
Senior Staff Specialist, Clinical Microbiology, ACT Pathology
Professor, School of Medicine, Australian National University

Acknowledgements

We would like to express our sincerest thanks to Dr Cecilia Li, Ms Grace Prael, Dr Shizar Nahidi and Dr Cristina Sotomayor-Castillo for their tremendously patient and dedicated assistance with gathering and analysing data, document management, proofing and the administration of this publication project.

We also extend our sincerest thanks to the Australasian College for Infection Prevention and Control and its members for their support of this publication, and to the many peer reviewers for their constructive feedback.

Ramon Z. Shaban
Brett G. Mitchell
Philip L. Russo
Deborough Macbeth

CHAPTER 1

Executive summary

Contents

Introduction—healthcare-associated infections in context

Healthcare–associated infections (HAIs) are a major patient safety problem. While research into infection prevention and control has led to improvements in our understanding of effective HAI prevention strategies, HAIs continue to occur and lead to morbidity, mortality and excess healthcare expenditure.[1,2] Central to all efforts to control and prevent HAIs is the inherent need to measure the burden of infection and disease, classically referred to as surveillance.

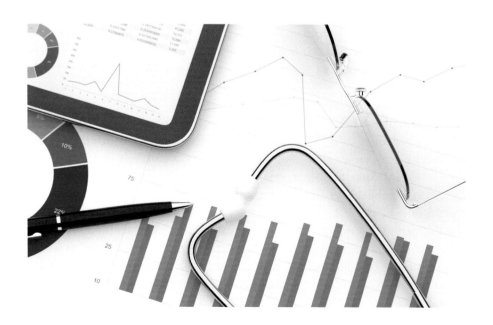

Australia is a federated country comprising of individual states and territories. The Australian healthcare system is a shared responsibility of the Australian Government and state and territory governments, and the responsibility of funding, policy development, regulation and service delivery is based on constitutional sovereignty. States and territories have sovereign constitution authority to deliver health services, and they each have their own health service organisation and system with different services, funding and management structures. The Australian, state and territory governments each contribute funding to public hospitals. Public hospitals are largely run and managed by state and territory governments through the local hospital networks (LHNs) and local health districts (LHDs), and they are responsible for the collection and management of healthcare information. There are currently 136 LHNs in Australia, of which 122 are geographically based and 14 are statewide or territory-wide networks.[3] State and territory governments license and regulate private hospitals that are owned by the private sector.

There is no single unified national HAI surveillance system because each Australian state and territory is responsible for, and administers, its own system. As such, there are different types of HAI epidemiological data being collected and reported in different ways across Australian jurisdictions. First, data on HAIs due to hospital-acquired complications (HACs)—a complication for which clinical risk mitigation strategies may reduce (but not necessarily eliminate) the risk of that complication occurring—are being collected. There are 16 different HAC categories (one of which is HAI-related) comprising of eight different HAI HAC types. Second, there are state-based systems for the surveillance and reporting of HAIs, but only some of these infections are reported. Third, data are published in the peer-reviewed and grey literature, which reports data from state and territory surveillance systems, as well as research into the epidemiology of HAI within Australian populations and groups. There has been no previously published report that collates these three datasets to report the epidemiology of HAIs in Australia.

This report is the first attempt to collate these publicly available surveillance data of HAI epidemiology in Australia. For the purposes of this monograph publicly available data is defined as data that is published electronically or in other forms and is freely available to the public. This report presents a collation and analysis of the three types of HAI data: 1. proportions of HAI HAC for the period 1 July 2017 to 30 June 2019; 2. publicly available Australian jurisdictional (state and territory) surveillance data for the period 2017 to 2019, where available; and 3. peer-reviewed literature data for the period 1 January 2010 to 31 August 2019. The methodology adopted by this report is documented in the Appendix (Chapter 10). For ease of presentation, the report is structured using the classification of HAIs according to the eight diagnoses within the HAI HAC established by the Australian Commission on Safety and Quality in Health Care.

Epidemiology of HAI in Australia by dataset

1. Healthcare-associated infection due to hospital-acquired complication (HAI HAC) data

Data on HAI HACs in Australia are collected by the Independent Hospital Pricing Authority (IHPA) but are not currently reported or publicly available. These data were provided upon request. The jurisdictions did not grant permission to publish the raw data but gave permission to report data by proportions. The number of HAI HACs are thus presented as a proportion. Data for each of the eight HAI diagnoses were provided but data regarding further subclass specifications and codes within each HAI diagnosis were not provided. The raw data from which these proportions were calculated were provided by IHPA (as per the methodology outlined in Chapter 10).[4]

The epidemiology of all HAI in Australian public hospitals (adult and paediatric) in proportions, as identified by HAC data, by state and territory for 2017–2018 is illustrated in Table 1.1 and Figure 1.1.

The epidemiology of all HAI in Australian public hospitals (as identified by HAC data) by state and territory for 2018–2019 is illustrated in Table 1.2 and Figure 1.2.

New South Wales, Victoria and Queensland are the most populous states in Australia. As such, approximately 75% to 80% of each reported HAI occurred in these three states. Proportions of each HAI in the majority of jurisdictions remained stable over the two reported time periods, with some notable exceptions. In Victoria,

Table 1.1 Nationwide distribution for all eight HAI HAC by jurisdiction (%), 1 July 2017 to 30 June 2018

HAI HAC	NSW	Vic.	Qld	SA	WA	Tas.	NT	ACT
Urinary tract infection	27.0	30.0	23.1	8.5	6.0	3.0	0.6	1.9
Surgical site infection	34.2	24.3	19.7	5.6	10.8	2.5	1.5	1.4
Pneumonia	28.2	29.6	17.2	12.1	6.8	2.9	1.1	2.1
Bloodstream infection	23.8	39.6	19.9	5.2	6.6	1.9	1.2	1.8
Central line and peripheral line associated bloodstream infection	41.0	17.8	21.0	4.5	10.7	2.0	1.1	1.8
Multi-resistant organism	29.2	30.6	21.7	5.3	7.9	2.2	1.4	1.6
Infection associated with prosthetics/implantable devices	31.8	19.4	26.4	9.1	7.4	2.2	2.0	1.6
Gastrointestinal infection	30.3	25.0	21.7	9.7	7.5	3.4	0.5	1.9

Note: NSW = New South Wales. Vic. = Victoria. Qld = Queensland. SA = South Australia. WA = Western Australia. Tas. = Tasmania. NT = Northern Territory. ACT = Australian Capital Territory. Data are proportions and totals for each jurisdiction may not equal 100% exactly due to rounding.
(Source: Compiled from IHPA data.)

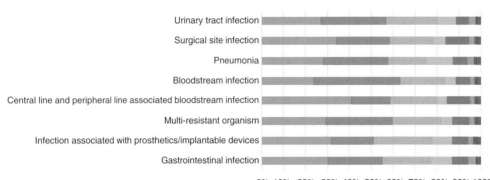

Figure 1.1 *Nationwide distribution for all eight HAI HAC by jurisdiction (%), 1 July 2017 to 30 June 2018*
Note: ACT = Australian Capital Territory. NSW = New South Wales. NT = Northern Territory. Qld = Queensland. SA = South Australia. Tas. = Tasmania. Vic. = Victoria. WA = Western Australia.
(Source: Compiled from IHPA data.)

Table 1.2 Nationwide distribution for all eight HAI HAC by jurisdiction (%), 1st July 2018 to 30th June 2019

HAI HAC	NSW	Vic.	Qld	SA	WA	Tas.	NT	ACT
Urinary tract infection	27.3	33.7	21.8	6.0	6.0	2.9	0.7	1.7
Surgical site infection	35.2	26.6	18.4	5.0	9.0	2.6	1.3	1.8
Pneumonia	28.2	32.7	16.0	10.2	6.4	3.1	1.3	2.1
Bloodstream infection	22.8	44.4	18.4	3.8	5.9	2.0	0.9	1.9
Central line and peripheral line associated bloodstream infection	38.4	18.6	22.7	5.0	9.6	3.0	0.7	2.1
Multi-resistant organism	28.3	33.6	20.3	4.2	7.6	2.6	1.4	1.9
Infection associated with prosthetics/implantable devices	33.6	23.2	22.3	7.9	7.6	2.4	1.4	1.6
Gastrointestinal infection	31.8	30.2	15.2	8.1	7.5	3.3	0.8	3.2

Note: ACT = Australian Capital Territory. NSW = New South Wales. NT = Northern Territory. Qld = Queensland. SA = South Australia. Tas. = Tasmania. Vic. = Victoria. WA = Western Australia. Data are proportions and totals for each jurisdiction may not equal 100% exactly due to rounding.
(Source: Compiled from IHPA data.)

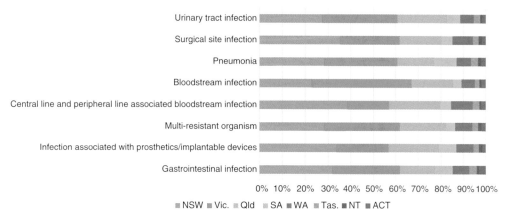

Figure 1.2 *Nationwide distribution for all eight HAI HAC by jurisdiction (%), 1 July 2018 to 30 June 2019*
Note: ACT = Australian Capital Territory. NSW = New South Wales. NT = Northern Territory. Qld = Queensland. SA = South Australia. Tas. = Tasmania. Vic. = Victoria. WA = Western Australia.
(Source: Compiled from IHPA data.)

reported bloodstream and gastrointestinal infections increased by 5% in 2018–2019. In Queensland, reported central line and peripheral line associated bloodstream infections and gastrointestinal infections decreased by 4% and 6.5%, respectively, in 2018–2019.

2. State and territory jurisdiction surveillance data

The only HAI for which data is publicly available from all jurisdictions is *Staphylococcus aureus* bacteraemia. There is no publicly available jurisdictional data for urinary tract infections or pneumonia. Victoria and Western Australia have publicly available data for six of the eight subcategories, while Tasmania has four and South Australia three. The remaining jurisdictions had no other HAI data available except for *Staphylococcus aureus* bacteraemia (Table 1.3).

Even when data is available within these categories from more than one jurisdiction, it is not always comparable. As an example, although surgical site infection data is available from both Victoria and Western Australia, there are differences in the type of surgical procedures where data is available; in those procedures for which data is available from both jurisdictions, they are stratified using different risk categories.

National *Staphylococcus aureus* bacteraemia rates were first published in 2010–2011, and are now a safety and quality indicator under the Australian Health Performance Framework.[5] A benchmark of 2.0 cases per 10,000 patient days was established, and in 2018–2019 all jurisdictions reported rates below the benchmark. This benchmark has since been reduced from 2.0 cases to 1.0 cases per 10,000 patient days. This is the only HAI that is reported nationally and by all jurisdictions.

Table 1.3 Jurisdictional publicly available data

HAI HAC	NSW	Vic.	Qld	SA	WA	Tas.	NT	ACT
Urinary tract infection	–	–	–	–	–	–	–	–
Surgical site infection	–	✓	–	–	✓	–	–	–
Pneumonia	–	–	–	–	–	–	–	–
Bloodstream infection	✓	✓	✓	✓	✓	✓	✓	✓
Central line and peripheral line associated bloodstream infection	–	✓	–	✓	✓	✓	–	–
Multi-resistant organism	–	✓	–	✓	✓	✓	–	–
Infection associated with prosthetics/implantable devices	–	✓	–	–	✓	–	–	–
Gastrointestinal infection	–	✓	–	–	✓	✓	–	–

Note: ✓ indicates that data is available. – indicates that data is unavailable. ACT = Australian Capital Territory. NSW = New South Wales. NT = Northern Territory. Qld = Queensland. SA = South Australia. Tas. = Tasmania. Vic. = Victoria. WA = Western Australia.
(Source: Compiled from IHPA data.)

3. Peer-reviewed literature data

The peer-reviewed literature reporting the incidence of HAIs in Australian hospitals is limited to specific infections, with considerable heterogeneity in methodological approaches and HAI definition, thus making it difficult to calculate the epidemiology of infection accurately. There have been two national point prevalence studies of HAI in Australia. The first in 1984 suggested that the overall adjusted prevalence of nosocomial (hospital-acquired) infection was 6.3% and the prevalence of community-acquired infection was 9.7%.[6] In 2008, the prevalence of HAIs in Australia was estimated to be about 200,000 HAIs, which proposed HAIs to be the most common complication affecting patients in hospital.[7] A 2017 systematic review of the burden of HAI in Australian hospitals suggested there were 83,096 HAIs per year in Australia, comprising 71,186 urinary tract infections, 4902 *Clostridium difficile* infections, 3946 surgical site infections, 1962 respiratory infections in acute stroke patients and 1100 hospital-onset *Staphylococcus aureus* bacteraemia HAIs.[1] The review noted this burden to be largely underestimated given the lack of or incomplete data on common infections such as pneumonia, gastroenterological and bloodstream infection, and suggested that the actual burden could be 50% to 60% higher. The second national point prevalence study of HAI in 2767 patients from 19 hospitals between August and November 2018 reported an overall HAI prevalence of adult acute inpatients with a HAI of 9.9% (363 HAIs in 273 patients; 95% CI: 8.8–11.0) ranging from 5.7% (95% CI: 2.9–11.0) to 17.0% (95% CI: 10.7–26.1). The most common HAIs were surgical site infection, pneumonia and urinary tract infection, comprising 64%

of all HAIs identified.[8] Multi-resistant organism (MRO) HAIs were documented for 10.3% of the patients. The HAI prevalence rate in this second study was higher than the previous Australian study, noting, however, the differences in methodologies that limit comparisons.

Synthesis and summary

This report presents original data and analyses documenting the epidemiology of HAIs in Australia. In Australia, at the time of writing, the publicly available HAI data depict a variable landscape with large sections uncharted. While there is considerable HAI surveillance data collected by Australian jurisdictions, limited data are published or made publicly available. There is a lack of standardised and systematic approaches to surveillance definitions and methodology. Recent research has demonstrated disparity between existing jurisdictional-based HAI surveillance activity. The peer-reviewed literature provides some additional data on the incidence of HAIs in Australian hospitals—albeit limited—making it difficult to calculate accurately the epidemiology of infection. It does, however, provide a limited view of the epidemiology of HAIs in Australian hospitals by using a variety of methods and definitions, which are sometimes unstated, in different populations. The recent introduction of hospital-acquired complications (HACs), a complication for which clinical risk mitigation strategies may reduce (but not necessarily eliminate) the risk of that complication occurring, has further added to the information that is gathered on HAIs in Australia, albeit not publicly reported. The proportions of HAI HACs, published in this report for the first time, provide some information regarding the burden of HAC-defined HAIs across Australian jurisdictions for 2017–2019. Results derived from HAC data are based on the interpretation of clinical records. They remain unvalidated. Furthermore, these HAC data represent the proportion of HAIs by state and territory and lack a numerator and denominator, and the procedures included in the data are undifferentiated in terms of procedure classification and infection type. The absence of a single national HAI surveillance system that includes, or takes into consideration, these data types, definitions and methodologies precludes an accurate estimate of the epidemiology and burden of HAIs in Australia.

References

1. Mitchell BG, Shaban RZ, Macbeth D, et al. The burden of healthcare-associated infection in Australian hospitals: A systematic review of the literature. *Infect Dis Health* 2017; **22**(3): 117–28.
2. National Healthcare Safety Network. Surveillance for Surgical Site Infection (SSI) Events. Atlanta: Centers for Disease Control; 2020.
3. Australian Commission on Safety and Quality in Health Care. AURA 2019: third Australian report on antimicrobial use and resistance in human health. Sydney: Australian Commission on Safety and Quality in Health Care, 2019.

4. Independent Hospital Pricing Authority. Healthcare-associated infections Hospital-acquired complication (HAI HAC) data. In: Independent Hospital Pricing Authority, editor. Sydney, Australia: Independent Hospital Pricing Authority; 2020.
5. Australian Institute of Health and Welfare. Bloodstream infections associated with hospital care 2018–19. Canberra: AIHW, 2020.
6. McLaws M-L, Gold J, Lirwing L, et al. The prevalence of nosocomial and community-acquired infections in Australian hospitals. *Med J Aust* 1984; **149**(11–12): 582–90.
7. Cruickshank M, Ferguson J, editors. Reducing harm to patients from healthcare-associated infection: the role of surveillance. Sydney, Australia: Australian Commission on Safety and Quality in Health Care; 2008.
8. Russo PL, Stewardson AJ, Cheng AC, et al. The prevalence of healthcare-associated infections among adult inpatients at nineteen large Australian acute-care public hospitals: a point prevalence survey. *Antimicrob Resist Infect Control* 2019; **8**: 114.

CHAPTER 2

Surgical site infection

Contents

Introduction

According to the World Health Organization (WHO), surgical site infection (SSI) is one of the most frequent types of healthcare–associated infection (HAI).[1] SSIs increase the length of hospital stay, add to the cost of healthcare and are associated with increased mortality.[2] In 2018, SSI data collected through the Centers for Disease Control and Prevention (CDC) National Healthcare Safety Network (NHSN) identified just over 21,000 surgical site infections following more than 2.8 million procedures

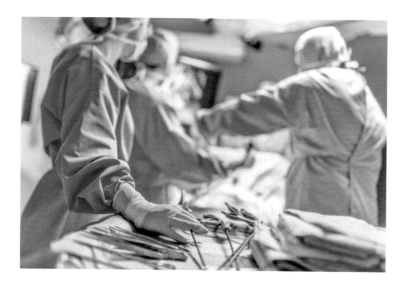

in participating acute-care hospitals in the United States. These data do not encompass all surgical procedures performed. Rather, they relate to a specific set of procedures included in the NHSN data collection program.[3]

There is no similar national surveillance program in Australia, and a set of standardised definitions is also lacking. However, a point prevalence survey conducted in 2018 identified that SSI was the most common HAI in the study cohort of 19 large acute-care hospitals.[4]

Efforts to reduce the risk of SSI have employed a range of strategies including but not limited to:[1,5,6]

- preoperative patient bathing with antimicrobial solutions
- preoperative skin preparation
- perioperative antibiotic prophylaxis
- glycaemic control
- clipping rather than shaving for body hair removal.

Ultimately, the effectiveness of any strategy—alone or in tandem—can only be determined through robust and systematic data collection. This chapter presents the publicly available Australian data on the incidence of SSI.

Definitions and context

The definition of an SSI varies, based on the classification of the wound (e.g. clean, clean-contaminated, contaminated, dirty) and the locus of infection (superficial, deep or organ/space). Some procedures involve more than one incision (e.g. coronary artery bypass graft [CABG]). Examples of SSI surveillance definitions are provided in Table 2.1. For further and more detailed explanations and their applications, please refer to the source document referenced.

This report presents a collation and analysis of the three types of Australian SSI data: 1. proportions of SSI hospital-acquired complication for the period 1 July 2017 to 30 June 2019; 2. publicly available state and territory jurisdiction surveillance data for the period 1 July 2017 to 30 June 2018; and 3. peer-reviewed literature data for the period 1 January 2010 to 31 August 2019. Each of these potential data sources were interrogated to gain insight into the incidence of SSI in Australia and the findings are presented on the following pages.

Findings

1. Healthcare-associated infection due to hospital-acquired complication (HAI HAC) data

Data on HAI HACs in Australia are collected by the Independent Hospital Pricing Authority (IHPA) but are not currently reported or publicly available.

Table 2.1 Examples of SSI surveillance definitions

Country/organisation	Subcategory	Overview of definition
Australia		No nationally agreed or defined surveillance definition.
United States CDC NHSN[7]★	Superficial incisional surgical site infection (SSI) (further definitions are provided in relation to primary incision site and secondary incision site)	Date of event occurs within 30 days after any NHSN operative procedure (where day 1 = the procedure date) **AND** involves skin and subcutaneous tissue of the incision **AND** patient has at least **_one_** of the following: a. purulent drainage from the superficial incision b. organism(s) identified from an aseptically obtained specimen from the superficial incision or subcutaneous tissue by a culture or non-culture-based microbiologic testing method which is performed for purposes of clinical diagnosis or treatment (e.g. not active surveillance culture/testing [ACT/AST]) c. superficial incision that is deliberately opened by a surgeon, physician★ or physician designee and culture or non-culture-based testing of the superficial incision or subcutaneous tissue is not performed **AND** patient has at least one of the following signs or symptoms: localised pain or tenderness; localised swelling; erythema; or heat d. diagnosis of a superficial incisional SSI by a physician★ or physician designee.

Continued

Table 2.1 Examples of SSI surveillance definitions—cont'd

Country/organisation	Subcategory	Overview of definition
	Deep incisional SSI (further definitions are provided in relation to deep primary incision site and deep secondary incision site)	The date of the event occurs within 30 or 90 days after the NHSN operative procedure (where day 1 = the procedure date) according to the list in Table 2 (where specific procedures are listed; see source document) **AND** involves deep soft tissues of the incision (for example fascia and muscle layers) **AND** patient has at least _**one**_ of the following: a. Purulent drainage from the deep incision. b. A deep incision that spontaneously dehisces, or is deliberately opened or aspirated by a surgeon, physician★ or physician designee **AND** organism(s) identified from the deep soft tissues of the incision by a culture or non-culture-based microbiologic testing method which is performed for purposes of clinical diagnosis or treatment (for example, not active surveillance culture/testing [ACT/AST]) or culture or non-culture-based microbiologic testing method is not performed; a culture or non-culture-based test from the deep soft tissues of the incision that has a negative finding does not meet this criterion **AND** patient has at least _**one**_ of the following signs or symptoms: fever (>38°C); localised pain or tenderness c. an abscess or other evidence of infection involving deep incision that is detected on gross anatomical or histopathologic exam, or imaging test.

Table 2.1 Examples of SSI surveillance definitions—cont'd

Country/organisation	Subcategory	Overview of definition
	Organ/space SSI	Date of event occurs within 30 or 90 days after the NHSN operative procedure (where day 1 = the procedure day) according to the list in Table 2 *[specific procedures are listed in the source document]* **AND** involves any part of the body deeper than the fascial muscle layers that is opened or manipulated during the operative procedure **AND** patient has at least **one** of the following: a. purulent drainage from a drain that is placed into the organ/space (e.g. closed suction drainage system, open drain, T-tube drain, CT-guided drainage) b. organism(s) identified from fluid or tissue in the organ/space by a culture or non-culture-based microbiologic testing method which is performed for the purposes of clinical diagnosis or treatment (e.g. not active surveillance culture/testing [ACT/AST]) c. an abscess or other evidence of infection involving the organ/space that is detected on gross anatomical or histopathologic exam, or imaging test evidence suggestive of infection **AND** meets at least **one** criterion for a specific organ/space infection site listed in Table 3 *[specific procedures are listed in the source document]*.

Continued

Table 2.1 Examples of SSI surveillance definitions—cont'd

Country/organisation	Subcategory	Overview of definition
Europe (ECDC)[8]	Superficial incisional	Infection occurs within 30 days after the operation and involves only skin and subcutaneous tissue of the incision and at least one of the following: • purulent drainage with or without laboratory confirmation, from the superficial incision • organisms isolated from an aseptically obtained culture of fluid or tissue from the superficial incision • at least one of the following signs or symptoms of infection: pain or tenderness, localised swelling, redness or heat and superficial incision is deliberately opened by surgeon, unless incision is culture-negative • diagnosis of superficial incisional SSI made by surgeon or attending physician.
	Deep incisional	Infection occurs within 30 days after the operation if no implant[†] is left in place or within 90 days if implant is in place and the infection appears to be related to the operation and infection involves deep soft tissue (e.g. fascia, muscle) of the incision and at least one of the following: • purulent drainage from the deep incision but not from the organ/space component of the surgical site • a deep incision spontaneously dehisces or is deliberately opened by a surgeon when the patient has at least one of the following signs or symptoms: fever (> 38°C), localised pain or tenderness, unless incision is culture-negative • an abscess or other evidence of infection involving the deep incision is found on direct examination, during reoperation or by histopathologic or radiologic examination • diagnosis of deep incisional SSI made by a surgeon or attending physician.

Table 2.1 Examples of SSI surveillance definitions—cont'd

Country/organisation	Subcategory	Overview of definition
	Organ/space	Infection occurs within 30 days after the operation if no implant[†] is left in place or 90 days if implant is in place and the infection appears to be related to the operation and infection involves any part of the anatomy (e.g. organs and spaces) other than the incision that was opened or manipulated during an operation and at least one of the following: • purulent discharge from a drain that is placed through a stab wound into the organ/space • organisms isolated from an aseptically obtained culture of fluid or tissue in the organ/space • an abscess or other evidence of infection involving the organ/space that is found on direct examination, during reoperation or by histopathologic or radiologic examination • diagnosis of organ/space SSI made by a surgeon or attending physician.

★ The term 'physician' for the purpose of application of the NHSN SSI criteria may be interpreted to mean a surgeon, infectious disease physician, emergency physician, other physician on the case or physician's designee (nurse practitioner or physician's assistant).

† The US National Nosocomial Infection Surveillance definition: a nonhuman-derived implantable foreign body (e.g. prosthetic heart valve, nonhuman vascular graft, mechanical heart or hip prosthesis) that is permanently placed in a patient during surgery.

Note: CDC = Centers for Disease Control. ECDC = European Centre for Disease Prevention and Control. NHSN = National Healthcare Safety Network.

These data were provided upon request. The jurisdictions did not grant permission to publish the raw data but gave permission to report data by proportions. The number of HAI HAC SSIs are thus presented as a proportion. The raw data from which these proportions were calculated were provided by the IHPA.[9]

SSIs in Australian public hospitals, as identified by HAI HAC data by state and territory for 2017–2018 and 2018–2019, are presented in Table 2.2 and Figure 2.1. New South Wales, Victoria and Queensland combined recorded 80% of Australia's proportion of SSIs over the two time periods. Proportions of SSI (%) in each jurisdiction remained stable.

2. Jurisdictional HAI data

The second potential source of data relating to SSI in Australian hospitals is from data published by the Australian state and territory health departments. A search of

Table 2.2 Nationwide distribution of HAC HAI SSIs by jurisdiction (%)

Jurisdiction	Timeframe	
	1 July 2017 – 30 June 2018	*1 July 2018 – 30 June 2019*
NSW	34.2	35.2
Vic.	24.3	26.6
Qld	19.7	18.4
SA	5.0	5.0
WA	10.8	9.0
Tas.	2.5	2.6
NT	1.5	1.3
ACT	1.4	1.8

Note: ACT = Australian Capital Territory. NSW = New South Wales. NT = Northern Territory. Qld = Queensland.
  SA = South Australia. Tas. = Tasmania. Vic. = Victoria. WA = Western Australia.
(Source: Compiled from IHPA data.)

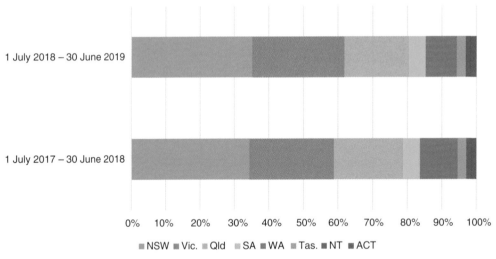

Figure 2.1 *Nationwide distribution of HAC HAI SSIs by jurisdiction (%)*
Note: ACT = Australian Capital Territory. NSW = New South Wales. NT = Northern Territory. Qld = Queensland. SA =
South Australia. Tas. = Tasmania. Vic. = Victoria. WA = Western Australia
(Source: Compiled from IHPA data.)

each jurisdictional website was undertaken to locate any data published on SSI. To
ensure accurate representation of the published data, each jurisdiction was contacted
and asked to provide the data collected and publicly available on a range of HAI
including SSI. The results of the searches and data provided on request are presented
in Table 2.3. Where data is not listed, data were not available.

Table 2.3 Publicly available jurisdictional SSI data for 2017–2018

Procedure	ACT	NSW	NT	Qld	SA	Tas.	Vic.[10]	WA[11]
Coronary artery bypass grafting (CABG)	–	–	–	–	–	–	2017–2018 Total infections. Low risk 2.8 ($n = 1574$) Higher risk 4.6 ($n = 583$)	–
Abdominal hysterectomy	–	–	–	–	–	–	2017–2018 Total infections. Low risk 0.6 ($n = 354$) Higher risk 0.4 ($n = 478$) Highest risk 0.5 ($n = 189$)	–
Caesarean section	–	–	–	–	–	–	2017–2018 Total infections. Low risk 0.4 ($n = 5384$) Higher risk 0.8 ($n = 4078$) Highest risk 1.6 ($n = 451$)	2017–2018 Total infections Risk all 1.32 ($n = 1436$) Risk index 0: 0.4 ($n = 4800$) Risk index 1: 0.59 ($n = 3038$) Risk index 2: 1.76 ($n = 626$) Risk index 3: 2.0 ($n = 50$)
Other cardiac surgery	–	–	–	–	–	–	2017–2018 Total infections. Low risk 1.0 ($n = 313$) Higher risk 2.4 ($n = 170$)	–

Continued

Table 2.3 Publicly available jurisdictional SSI data for 2017–2018—cont'd

Procedure	ACT	NSW	NT	Qld	SA	Tas.	Vic.[10]	WA[11]
Hip replacement/ hip arthroplasty	–	–	–	–	–	–	2017–2018 Total infections. Low risk 0.6 ($n = 354$) Higher risk 0.4 ($n = 478$) Highest risk 0.5 ($n = 189$)	2017–2018 Total infections Risk all: 0.63 ($n = 315$) Risk index 0: 0.54 ($n = 2600$) Risk index 1: 0.89 ($n = 1682$) Risk index 2: 2.74 ($n = 219$) Risk index 3: 0 ($n = 17$)
Knee replacement/ knee arthroplasty	–	–	–	–	–	–	2017–2018 Total infections. Low risk 2.8 ($n = 1574$) Higher risk 4.6 ($n = 583$)	2017–2018 Total infections Risk all: 0.8 ($n = 377$) Risk index 0: 0.43 ($n = 3708$) Risk index 1: 0.64 ($n = 2671$) Risk index 2: 1.77 ($n = 451$) Risk index 3: 10.0 ($n = 20$)
Colorectal surgery	–	–	–	–	–	–	2017–2018 Total infections. Lowest risk 3.2 ($n = 189$) Low risk 3.7 ($n = 656$) Higher risk 5.1 ($n = 838$) Highest risk 10.8 ($n = 189$)	–

Table 2.3 Publicly available jurisdictional SSI data for 2017–2018—cont'd

Procedure	ACT	NSW	NT	Qld	SA	Tas.	Vic.[10]	WA[11]
Risk index definitions	–	–	–	–	–	–	Lowest risk: undefined Low risk: undefined Higher risk: undefined Highest risk: undefined	Risk stratification is based on the CDC NHSN (United States) risk index. Risk 'All' applies to HISWA hospitals that perform fewer than 100 procedures annually and are not required to assign a risk index score. Procedure type: primary and revision.

Note: – indicates that data was not available. ACT = Australian Capital Territory. CDC = Centers for Disease Control. HISWA = Healthcare Infection Surveillance Western Australia. NHSN = National Healthcare Safety Network. NSW = New South Wales. NT = Northern Territory. Qld = Queensland. SA = South Australia. Tas. = Tasmania. Vic. = Victoria. WA = Western Australia.

3. Peer-reviewed literature data

The final data source for Australian SSI is the peer-reviewed literature. The findings from articles identified in the peer-reviewed literature are summarised in Table 2.4. Ten articles were found that report on surgical wound infection incidence or prevalence. Of these, one study reported on SSI from all states and territories (except the Northern Territory), three studies reported on SSI in New South Wales, two each on SSI in Victoria and Western Australia, and one each on SSI in Queensland and South Australia. There were no studies identified reporting on SSI in the Northern Territory.

Infection definitions used in the studies varied and included no stated definition, established definitions such as those described earlier from CDC NHSN and the European Centre for Disease Prevention and Control (ECDC). Some studies identified infections based on the ICD-10-AM/ACHI/ACS derived from patient records.[4,12–19] Due to variation between study methods, population groups, comparison of surgical procedures and definitions is not possible.

Table 2.4 Data on SSIs identified from literature research

Lead author	Year	Location (no. of hospitals)	Year(s) study was undertaken	Population	Type of HAI monitored	Key finding
Austin[12]	2017	NSW (1)	2011–2014	98 ECMO patients	Wound	20 per 1000 ECMO days
Bagheri[13]	2017	NSW (?)	2002–2013	58,096 surgical patients	SSIs (colorectal)	9.64% (95% CI: 9.40–9.88)
Betts[14]	2019	Qld (?)	2009–2015	All inpatient live births in Qld in study period	Surgical wound infection	0.37%
Chandrananth[15]	2016	Vic. (3)	2011–2014	1019 patients undergoing hip or knee arthroplasty	SSI	Total SSI rate was 2.7%; rate of 1.7% in those adherent to antibiotic guidelines, versus 5.0% if non-adherent
Furuya–Kanamori[16]	2017	NSW (?)	2002–2013	Adult patients who underwent colorectal, joint replacement, spinal or cardiac procedures in a public hospital. Number of procedures included: 58,096 colorectal; 113,123 joint replacement; 26,694 spinal; 39,274 cardiac.	SSIs (joint replacement, colorectal, spinal and cardiac operations)	9.64% (95% CI: 9.40–9.88) SSI for colorectal 3.33% (95% CI: 3.23–3.44) for joint replacement 2.33% (95% CI: 2.15–2.52) for spinal 5.66% (95% CI: 5.43–5.89) for cardiac

Jarratt[17]	2013	SA (1)	2003–2011	All hospital	SSI	MRO: 57 (55.3%); non-MRO: 602 (65.9%)
Kelly[18]	2017	WA (1)	2000–2002, 2010–2012	184 patients who underwent MLLA: 87 in 2000–2002, 97 in 2010–2012	WIs	2000–2002: 23/87 2010–2012: 12/97
Lavers[19]	2018	WA (1)	2015–2017	250 patients (male/female) who underwent breast procedures	SSIs	5.2% (13/250)
Russo[4]	2019	All states/territories except NT (19)	2018	2767 acute adult inpatients	SSI	SSIs: 3.6% (95% CI: 2.9–4.4)
Tao[20]	2015	Vic. (1)	2012 (1 month)	88 orthopaedic patients (95 surgeries)	SSI	7/88 patients (7%) patients developed an SSI; 6/7 = superficial infection, 1/7 deep peri-prosthetic infection

Note: ECMO = extracorporeal membrane oxygenation. HAI = healthcare-associated infection. MLLA = major lower limb amputation. MRO = multi-resistant organism. NSW = New South Wales. NT = Northern Territory. Qld = Queensland. SA = South Australia. SSI = surgical site infection. Vic. = Victoria. WA = Western Australian. W1 = wound infection.

Table 2.5 Other related data identified from literature research

Lead author	Year	Location	Year(s) study was undertaken	Population	Type of HAI monitored	Key finding
Jarratt[17]	2013	SA (1)	2003–2011	All hospital	Skin or soft tissue infection	MRO: 5 (4.9%); non-MRO: 2 (0.2%)

Note: MRO = multi-resistant organism. SA = South Australia.

The study by Jarratt[17] focused on the relationship between patient characteristics and the development of a multi-resistant organism HAI considering all infection sites. In this study conducted in South Australia, 55% of the infections identified had the surgical site listed as the primary site of infection with the multi-resistant organism (Table 2.5).

The definition of HAI applied in each of the studies identified in the literature are listed in Table 2.6.

Synthesis and summary

Surgical site infection is reported to have the greatest impact on hospital length of stay and yet public SSI data are only available in two of the Australian jurisdictions: Victoria and Western Australia. Both states used the same definitions (CDC NHSN)[7] and both reported on SSI in total hip arthroplasty, total knee arthroplasty and caesarean section. The Victorian program included additional procedures.

Results derived from HAC data are based on the interpretation of clinical records. They remain unvalidated. Furthermore, these data as they have been provided represent the proportion of infections by state and territory and lack a numerator and denominator, and the procedures included in the data are undifferentiated in terms of procedure classification and infection type.

The peer-reviewed literature does provide more detailed information; however, the variety of methods used, definitions applied (or not stated) and target populations provides a fractured view of SSI in Australian hospitals. The point prevalence survey provides the most consistent approach and highlights SSI as the most frequent of all the HAI included in the study.

In Australia, at the time of writing, the publicly available data on SSI depict a variable landscape with large sections uncharted. It is difficult, if not impossible, to develop and implement rational infection prevention strategies without baseline measurement of the current situation. Only then can strategies be tested and their impact measured. This requires a standardised and systematic approach to surveillance definitions and methodology.

Table 2.6 HAI definitions used in the identified studies

Lead author	Year	HAI definition used
Austin[12]	2017	WIs: used CDC NHSN criteria for superficial incisional SSI or skin/soft tissue infection; classified as ECMO–related if occurred on site of a non-healed cannulation wound, or were believed to be related to wound—regardless of time since ECMO cannula removal. Sternal WIs: CDC NHSN criteria for deep incisional or organ/space SSI.
Bagheri[13]	2017	'Infection following a surgical procedure' code (ICD-10-AM T81.4) associated with colorectal surgeries was used for the study. Codes obtained from Admitted Patient Data Collection for patients aged 18+.
Betts[14]	2019	'Obstetric surgical wound infection' code ICD-10-AM O86
Chandrananth[15]	2016	CDC definition of SSI
Furuya-Kanamori[16]	2017	'Infection following a surgical procedure' code ICD-10-AM T81.4 and 'infection due to prosthetic device, implants and grafts' codes ICD-10-AM T82.6-T82.7, T83.5-T83.6, T84.5-T84.7, T85.7
Jarratt[17]	2013	CDC definition of SSI
Kelly[18]	2017	None
Lavers[19]	2018	None
Russo[4]	2019	ECDC definition of SSI
Tao[22]	2015	CDC NHSN definition of SSIs, which is also used by VICNISS; nine SSIs were defined as infections occurring 'following an operative procedure (with) no evidence that the infection was present or incubating at the time of the hospital admission'; four wound classifications were in accord with the National Academy of Science (United States) classification.

Note: WI = wound infection. CDC = Centers for Disease Control and Prevention. NHSN = National Healthcare Safety Network. ECMO = extracorporeal membrane oxygenation. ICD = International Classification of Diseases. ECDC = European Centre for Disease Prevention and Control. VICNISS = Victorian Nosocomial Infection Surveillance System.

References

1. World Health Organization. Global guidelines for the prevention of surgical site infection. Second Edn. Geneva: World Health Organization; 2018.
2. Bull A, McGechie D, Richards M, et al. Surgical site infection. In: Cruickshank M, Ferguson J, eds. Reducing harm to patients from healthcare associated infection: The role of surveillance. Canberra: Australian Commission on Safety and Quality in Health Care; 2008.

3. National Healthcare Safety Network. Current HAI Progress Report: 2018 National and State Healthcare-Associated Infections Progress Report. 2018 National and State HAI Progress Report SIR Data—Acute Care Hospitals. Atlanta: Centers for Disease Control and Prevention; 2018.

4. Russo PL, Stewardson AJ, Cheng AC, et al. The prevalence of healthcare-associated infections among adult inpatients at nineteen large Australian acute-care public hospitals: a point prevalence survey. *Antimicrob Resist Infect Control* 2019; **8**: 114.

5. Berrios-Torres SI, Umscheid CA, Bratzler DW, et al. Centers for Disease Control and Prevention Guideline for the Prevention of Surgical Site Infection, 2017. *JAMA Surg* 2017; **152**(8): 784–91.

6. National Institute for Health and Care Excellence. NICE Guideline [NG125]: Surgical site infections: prevention and treatment. London: National Institute for Health and Care Excellence; 2019.

7. National Healthcare Safety Network. Surveillance for Surgical Site Infection (SSI) Events. Atlanta: Centers for Disease Control; 2020.

8. European Centre for Disease Prevention and Control. Surveillance of surgical site infections and prevention indicators in European hospitals—HAISSI protocol. Solna: European Centre for Disease Prevention and Control; 2017.

9. Independent Hospital Pricing Authority. Healthcare-associated infections Hospital-acquired complication (HAI HAC) data. In: Independent Hospital Pricing Authority, editor. Sydney, Australia: Independent Hospital Pricing Authority; 2020.

10. Department of Health and Human Services, The University of Melbourne, The Royal Melbourne Hospital, The Peter Doherty Institute for Infection and Immunity. Healthcare-associated infection in Victoria: Surveillance report for 2016–17 and 2017–18. Melbourne, Australia, 2018.

11. Communicable Disease Control Directorate. Healthcare Infection Surveillance Western Australia: Annual Report 2017–18. Perth, Western Australia, 2018.

12. Austin DE, Kerr SJ, Al-Soufi S, et al. Nosocomial infections acquired by patients treated with extracorporeal membrane oxygenation. *Crit Care Resusc* 2017; **19**(Suppl 1): 68–75.

13. Bagheri N, Furuya-Kanamori L, Doi SAR, et al. Geographical outcome disparities in infection occurrence after colorectal surgery: An analysis of 58,096 colorectal surgical procedures. *Int J Surg* 2017; **44**: 117–21.

14. Betts KS, Kisely S, Alati R. Predicting common maternal postpartum complications: leveraging health administrative data and machine learning. *BJOG* 2019; **126**(6): 702–9.

15. Chandrananth J, Rabinovich A, Karahalios A, et al. Impact of adherence to local antibiotic prophylaxis guidelines on infection outcome after total hip or knee arthroplasty. *J Hosp Infect* 2016; **93**(4): 423–7.

16. Furuya-Kanamori L, Doi SAR, Smith PN, et al. Hospital effect on infections after four major surgical procedures: outlier and volume-outcome analysis using all-inclusive state data. *J Hosp Infect* 2017; **97**(2): 115–21.

17. Jarratt LS, Miller ER. The relationship between patient characteristics and the development of a multi-resistant healthcare-associated infection in a private South Australian hospital. *Healthc Inf* 2013; **18**: 94–101.

18. Kelly DA, Pedersen S, Tosenovsky P, et al. Major Lower Limb Amputation: Outcomes are Improving. *Ann Vasc Surg* 2017; **45**: 29–34.

19. Lavers A, Yip WS, Sunderland B, et al. Surgical antibiotic prophylaxis use and infection prevalence in non-cosmetic breast surgery procedures at a tertiary hospital in Western Australia—a retrospective study. *PeerJ* 2018; **6**: e5724.

20. Tao P, Marshall C, Bucknill A. Surgical site infection in orthopaedic surgery: an audit of perioperative practice at a tertiary centre. *Healthc Inf* 2015; **20**(2): 39–45.

CHAPTER 3

Urinary tract infection

Contents

Introduction

Point prevalence studies conducted in Europe, the United States and Australia all suggest that urinary tract infections (UTIs) are common healthcare-associated infections (HAIs) in hospitals.[1–3] Approximately 20% of HAIs are UTIs.[1–3] Healthcare–associated

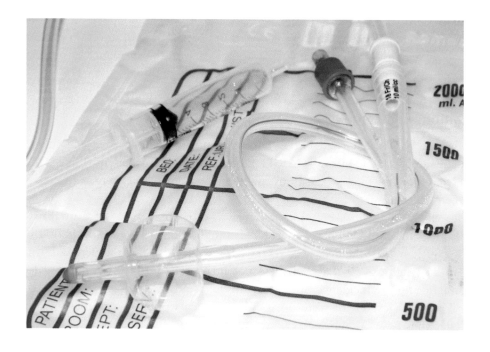

UTIs contribute to increased length of stay in hospitals and are associated with morbidity and mortality.[4] In Australia, there are an estimated 380,000 hospital bed days lost annually to healthcare-associated UTIs.[4] Antimicrobial resistance also poses increasing challenges for UTI treatment.[5,6]

Urinary catheter use is often associated with UTIs. The vast proportion of UTIs are catheter-associated UTIs (CAUTIs).[7] An Australian point prevalence study not only demonstrated a high proportion of UTIs being CAUTIs, but identified that 26% of patients surveyed across six hospitals had a urinary catheter during their stay (period prevalence).[7] These data are consistent with incidence data from the United Kingdom, suggesting that 13% of hospitalised patients receive a catheter.[8] Indwelling urinary catheters are inserted unnecessarily and remain in place longer than necessary.[9] These are two important risk factors for CAUTI and allow for targeted interventions to reduce incidence.[10–12]

The association between indwelling urinary catheter use and UTIs does provide a strong rationale for a program to prevent CAUTI. Prevention measures to date have focused on five main areas:

1. assessing the need for urinary catheter use in the first instance (prevention of inappropriate catheter use)
2. correct insertion practices
3. appropriate maintenance of urinary catheters
4. prompt removal of urinary catheters
5. surveillance (and feedback) of process or outcome measures related to CAUTI and UTIs.[10–15]

The last element described, surveillance, is the cornerstone of infection prevention and control activities. In this chapter, Australian data on the incidence of healthcare-associated UTIs, including CAUTIs, are presented.

Definitions and context

The definition of a UTI and CAUTI is a potentially complex area and subject to debate. Examples of UTI and CAUTI definitions are provided in Table 3.1. For further and more detailed explanations and their applications, please refer to the source document referenced.

This chapter presents a collation and analysis of the two types of Australian UTI data: 1. proportions of UTI hospital-acquired complication (HAC) for the period 1 July 2017 to 30 June 2019; and 2. peer-reviewed literature data for the period 1 January 2010 to 31 August 2019. Each of these potential data sources were interrogated to gain insight into the incidence of UTI in Australia and the findings are presented on the following pages. There were no jurisdictional data publicly available for urinary tract infections.

Table 3.1 Examples of UTI surveillance definitions

Country/ organisation	Subcategory	Overview of definition
Australia	UTI and CAUTI	No nationally agreed or defined surveillance definition.
United States (CDC NHSN[16]★†)	Symptomatic urinary tract infection (SUTI)	Patient must meet conditions 1, 2 and 3 below. 1. Patient had an indwelling urinary catheter that had been in place for more than 2 consecutive days in an inpatient location on the date of event AND was either: • present for any portion of the calendar day on the date of event OR • removed the day before the date of event. 2. Patient has at least one of the following signs or symptoms: fever (> 38.0°C), suprapubic tenderness, costovertebral angle pain or tenderness, urinary urgency, urinary frequency or dysuria. 3. Patient has a urine culture with no more than two species of organisms identified, at least one of which is a bacterium of $\geq 10^5$ CFU/mL.
	Asymptomatic bacteraemic UTI (ABUTI)	Patient must meet conditions 1, 2 and 3 below. 1. Patient with or without an indwelling urinary catheter has no signs or symptoms of SUTI 1 or 2 according to age. 2. Patient has a urine culture with no more than two species of organisms identified, at least one of which is a bacterium of $\geq 10^5$ CFU/mL. 3. Patient has organism identified from blood specimen with at least one matching bacterium to the bacterium at > 100,000 CFU/mL identified in the urine specimen, or is eligible criterion 2 (without fever) and matching common commensal(s) in the urine. All elements of the ABUTI criterion must occur during the infection window period.

Continued

Table 3.1 Examples of UTI surveillance definitions—cont'd

Country/organisation	Subcategory	Overview of definition
	Urinary system infection (USI)	Other infections of the urinary system must meet at least one of the following criteria. 1. Patient has organisms identified from fluid (excluding urine) or tissue from affected site. 2. Patient has an abscess or other evidence of infection on gross anatomical exam, during invasive procedure, or on histopathologic exam. 3. Patient has at least one of the following signs or symptoms: fever (> 38.0°C), localised pain or tenderness, and at least one of the following: (a) purulent drainage from affected site; (b) organisms identified from blood and imaging test evidence of infection (e.g. ultrasound, CT scan, magnetic resonance imaging [MRI] or radiolabel scan [gallium, technetium]) which if equivocal is supported by clinical correlation (i.e. physician documentation of antimicrobial treatment for urinary system infection). 4. Patient < 1 year of age has at least one of the following signs or symptoms: fever (> 38.0°C), hypothermia (< 36.0°C), apnoea, bradycardia, lethargy, vomiting, and at least one of the following: (a) purulent drainage from affected site; or (b) organisms identified from blood and imaging test evidence of infection (e.g. ultrasound, CT scans, MRI or radiolabel scan [gallium, technetium]).
	CAUTI	A UTI where an indwelling urinary catheter was in place for more than 2 consecutive days in an inpatient location on the date of event, with day of device placement being Day 1, AND an indwelling urinary catheter was in place on the date of the event or the day before. If an indwelling urinary catheter was in place for more than 2 consecutive days in an inpatient location and then removed, the date of event for the UTI must be the day of device discontinuation or the next day for the UTI to be catheter-associated.

Table 3.1 Examples of UTI surveillance definitions—cont'd

Country/ organisation	Subcategory	Overview of definition
Europe (ECDC point prevalence definition[17†‡])	UTI-A: microbiologically confirmed symptomatic UTI	• Patient has at least one of the following signs or symptoms with no other recognised cause: fever (> 38°C), urgency, frequency, dysuria or suprapubic tenderness AND • patient has a positive urine culture (i.e. ≥ 10^5 microorganisms per mL of urine with no more than two species of microorganisms.
	UTI-B: not microbiologically confirmed symptomatic UTI	• Patient has at least two of the following with no other recognised cause: fever (> 38°C), urgency, frequency, dysuria or suprapubic tenderness AND • at least one of the following: positive dipstick for leucocyte esterase and/or nitrate; pyuria urine specimen with ≥ 10 WBC/mL or ≥ 3 WBC/high power field of unspun urine; organisms seen on Gram stain of unspun urine; at least two urine cultures with repeated isolation of the same uropathogen (Gram-negative bacteria or *Staphylococcus saprophyticus*) with ≥ 10^2 colonies/mL urine in non-voided specimens; ≤ 10^5 colonies/mL of a single uropathogen (Gram-negative bacteria or *Staphylococcus saprophyticus*) in a patient being treated with an effective antimicrobial agent for a urinary infection; physician diagnosis of a urinary tract infection; physician institutes appropriate therapy for a urinary infection.

Continued

Table 3.1 Examples of UTI surveillance definitions—cont'd

Country/ organisation	Subcategory	Overview of definition

	UTI-C: asymptomatic bacteriuria: EXCLUDED FOR PPS, not to be reported*	• Patient has no fever (i.e. temp is < 38°C), urgency, frequency, dysuria or suprapubic tenderness and either of the following criteria:
		  ○ patient has had an indwelling urinary catheter within 7 days before urine is cultured
		  AND
		  ○ patient has a urine culture (i.e. ≥ 10^5 microorganisms per mL of urine) with no more than two species of microorganisms; patient has not had an indwelling urinary catheter within 7 days before the first positive culture
		  AND
		  ○ patient has had at least two positive urine cultures ≥ 10^5 microorganisms per mL of urine with repeated isolation of the same microorganism and no more than two species of microorganisms.

*Please refer to original source for additional details, including but not limited to criteria for different age groups, subclassifications of SUTI and criteria for signs and symptoms. Also required to meet definition of HAI using the defined window periods.[18]

†also required to meet the definition of healthcare associated. Day 3 onwards; OR day 1 or day 2 AND patient discharged from acute care hospital in preceding 48 hours; OR day 1 or day 2 AND patient has relevant device inserted on this admission prior to onset.

‡Abbreviated version; refer to source document for full details.

Note: CDC = Centers for Disease Control. ECDC = European Centre for Disease Prevention and Control. NHSN = National Healthcare Safety Network.

Findings

1. Healthcare-associated infection due to hospital-acquired complication (HAI HAC) data

Data on HAI HACs in Australia are collected by the Independent Hospital Pricing Authority (IHPA) but are not currently reported or publicly available. These data were provided upon request. The jurisdictions did not grant permission to publish the raw data but gave permission to report data by proportions. The number of HAI HAC UTIs are thus presented as a proportion. The raw data from which these proportions were calculated were provided by the IHPA.[19]

The burden of UTI in Australian public hospitals by proportion, as identified by HAI HAC data, by state and territory for 2017–2018 and 2018–2019 is presented in Table 3.2 and Figure 3.1. Over the two time periods, 80% of reported UTIs

Table 3.2 Nationwide distribution of HAC HAI UTIs by jurisdiction (%)

Jurisdiction	Timeframe	
	1 July 2017 – 30 June 2018	*1 July 2018 – 30 June 2019*
NSW	27.0	27.3
Vic.	30.0	33.7
Qld	23.1	21.8
SA	8.5	6.0
WA	6.0	6.0
Tas.	3.0	2.9
NT	0.6	0.7
ACT	1.9	1.7

Note: ACT = Australian Capital Territory. NSW = New South Wales. NT = Northern Territory. Qld = Queensland. SA = South Australia. Tas. = Tasmania. Vic. = Victoria. WA = Western Australia.
(Source: Compiled from IHPA data.)

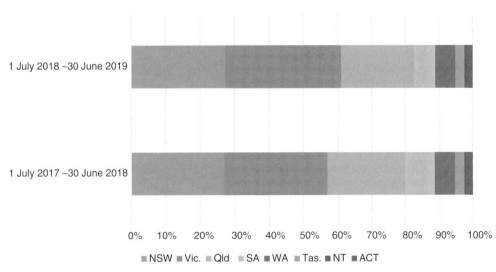

Figure 3.1 *Nationwide distribution of HAC HAI UTIs by jurisdiction (%)*
Note: ACT = Australian Capital Territory. NSW = New South Wales. NT = Northern Territory. Qld = Queensland.
SA = South Australia. Tas. = Tasmania. Vic. = Victoria. WA = Western Australia.
(Source: Compiled from IHPA data.)

occurred in New South Wales, Victoria and Queensland (the most populous states). Proportions of UTIs (%) in each jurisdiction were generally consistent across the time periods.

2. Jurisdictional healthcare-associated infection data

No data from jurisdictions on the surveillance on UTI or CAUTI was identified.

3. Peer-reviewed data

Table 3.3 summarises the findings from articles identified from the peer-reviewed literature. Six articles that describe the incidence or prevalence of UTIs (including CAUTIs) are listed. Two studies were conducted in Victoria,[20,21] with one study each in New South Wales,[4] South Australia[22] and Western Australia[23]. One study was conducted in multiple jurisdictions.[3] There were no studies identified from the Northern Territory. Studies used a variety of definitions to define a case of UTI, examples of which are provided in Table 3.4. There was heterogeneity of the studies with respect to population groups, design, outcome measures and definitions used. For these reasons, pooling of data was not possible. Two of the larger studies, one conducted in two intensive care units over a 6-year period,[20] the other in eight hospitals over a 4.5-year period,[4] found a similar incidence of UTI: 1.4% and 1.7% per patient admission, respectively. A point prevalence study conducted in 19 Australian hospitals found a point prevalence of 2.4%,[3] consistent with point prevalence studies conducted internationally.[1,2]

Synthesis and summary

Despite UTIs being one of the most common HAIs acquired in hospital, at the time of data collection, no Australian state or territory currently had publicly available data on the frequency of UTIs, including CAUTIs. HAC data does collect coding data for UTIs. However, coding data for UTIs has been shown to be consistently unreliable.[24,25] The distribution of the burden of UTI HAC data across the country, as presented in Table 3.2 and Figure 3.1, potentially reflects hospital activity and/or population. However, as we were unable to publish numerator or denominator data for HAC data, interpretation of these data is not possible.

Evaluation of interventions to reduce UTI and CAUTI using UTI HAC data is difficult, given the availability and variability of these data. An important element of informing and improving practice is timely, specific feedback. Both peer-reviewed data and HAC data have limitations in this regard. At this point in time in Australia, the clearest picture of the burden of UTIs comes from the peer-reviewed literature. However, these data are limited by publication bias, as well as challenges interpreting data from studies that use different approaches and case definitions of UTI.

Table 3.3 Data on urinary tract infections identified from literature research

Lead author	Year	Location (no. of hospitals)	Year(s) study was undertaken	Population	Type of HAI monitored	Key finding
Aubron[20]	2017	Vic. (2)	2008–2013	ICU patients (compared platelet transfusion recipients to non–platelet transfusion recipients)	Bacteriuria	All patients: 1.4% (262/18,965) Platelet transfusion recipients: 4% (89/2250) Non-platelet transfusion recipients: 1% (173/16,715)
Goodes[23]	2019	WA (1)	2015–2017	Traumatic spinal cord injury patients	UTI	61.4% (43/70) experienced one or more UTIs during admission
Jarratt[22]	2013	SA (1)	2003–2011	All hospital	UTI	MRO UTI: 30.1% (31/103) Non-MRO UTI: 5.9% (54/914)
Mitchell[4]	2016	NSW (8)	2010–2014	All hospital	HAUTI	1.73% (2821/162,503) (95% CI: 1.67–1.80)
Roth[21]	2015	Vic. (311)	2007–2012	TRUS biopsy patients and were readmitted within 7 days for infective complications	Infective complication of TRUS biopsy (systemic or UTI)	UTI 0.8% (279/34,865) All infective complication: 1.73% (604/34,865) (95% CI: 1.63–1.92%)
Russo[3]	2019	All states/ territories except NT (19)	2018	2767 acute adult inpatients	UTI	UTI: 2.4% (66/2767) (95% CI: 1.9–3.0)

Note: HAI = healthcare-associated infection. HAUTI = healthcare-associated urinary tract infection. ICU = intensive care unit. MRO = multi-resistant organism. NSW = New South Wales. NT = Northern Territory. Qld = Queensland. SA = South Australia. TRUS = transrectal ultrasound-guided. UTI = urinary tract infection. Vic. = Victoria. WA = Western Australia.

Table 3.4 HAI definitions used in the identified studies

Lead author	Year	HAI definition used
Aubron[20]	2017	Infection = bacteraemia or bacteriuria occurring in ICU after 48 hours of ICU stay
Goodes[23]	2019	UTI = bacteriuria (as defined by positive culture with minimum CFU requirement) with presence of symptomatology, as defined by Infectious Diseases Society of America's 2009 International Clinical Practice Guidelines
Jarratt[22]	2013	Defined as any localised or systemic condition resulting from an infectious agent or toxin for which no evidence was apparent on admission to the acute care setting
Mitchell[4]	2016	HAUTI considered present when patients had a positive urine culture more than 2 days after admission, according to the following criteria: positive for at least one species of Enterobacteriaceae, > 105/mL of urine, and no more than two species of microorganisms; a healthcare-associated bacteraemia secondary to HAUTI was defined as a positive blood culture occurring in a patient hospitalised > 48 hours, where the source was the urinary tract; multi-resistance was defined as an organism resistant to three or more of amoxicillin potassium clavulanate, ceftriaxone, gentamicin, trimethoprim or norfloxacin
Roth[21]	2015	International Classification of Disease (ICD-10-AM)
Russo[3]	2019	European Centre for Disease Prevention and Control

Note: CFU = colony forming units. HAI = healthcare-associated infection. HAUTI = hospital-acquired urinary tract infection. ICU = intensive care unit. UTI = urinary tract infection.

References

1. Magill SS, Edwards JR, Bamberg W, et al. Multistate point-prevalence survey of health care–associated infections. *N Engl J Med* 2014; **370**(13): 1198–208.
2. European Centre for Disease Prevention and Control. Point prevalence survey of healthcare-associated infections and antimicrobial use in European acute care hospitals. Stockholm: European Centre for Disease Prevention and Control; 2013.
3. Russo PL, Stewardson AJ, Cheng AC, et al. The prevalence of healthcare-associated infections among adult inpatients at nineteen large Australian acute-care public hospitals: a point prevalence survey. *Antimicrob Resist Infect Control* 2019; **8**: 114.
4. Mitchell BG, Ferguson JK, Anderson M, et al. Length of stay and mortality associated with healthcare-associated urinary tract infections: a multi-state model. *J Hosp Infect* 2016; **93**(1): 92–9.
5. Fasugba O, Mitchell BG, Mnatzaganian G, et al. Five-year antimicrobial resistance patterns of urinary *Escherichia coli* at an Australian tertiary hospital: time series analyses of prevalence data. *PLoS ONE* 2016; **11**(10): e0164306.
6. Fasugba O, Gardner A, Mitchell BG, et al. Ciprofloxacin resistance in community- and hospital-acquired *Escherichia coli* urinary tract infections: a systematic review and meta-analysis of observational studies. *BMC Infect Dis* 2015; **15**(1): 545.
7. Gardner A, Mitchell B, Beckingham W, et al. A point prevalence cross-sectional study of healthcare-associated urinary tract infections in six Australian hospitals. *BMJ Open* 2014; **4**(7): e005099.

8. Shackley DC, Whytock C, Parry G, et al. Variation in the prevalence of urinary catheters: a profile of National Health Service patients in England. *BMJ Open* 2017; **7**(6): e013842.

9. Meddings J, Rogers MA, Macy M, et al. Systematic review and meta-analysis: reminder systems to reduce catheter-associated urinary tract infections and urinary catheter use in hospitalized patients. *Clin Infect Dis* 2010; **51**(5): 550–60.

10. Lo E, Nicolle L, Classen D, et al. Strategies to prevent catheter-associated urinary tract infections in acute care hospitals. *Infect Control Hosp Epidemiol* 2008; **29 Suppl 1**(S1): S41–50.

11. Meddings J, Rogers MA, Krein SL, et al. Reducing unnecessary urinary catheter use and other strategies to prevent catheter-associated urinary tract infection: an integrative review. *BMJ Qual Saf* 2014; **23**(4): 277–89.

12. Mitchell BG, Northcote M, Cheng AC, et al. Reducing urinary catheter use using an electronic reminder system in hospitalized patients: A randomized stepped-wedge trial. *Infect Control Hosp Epidemiol* 2019; **40**(4): 427–31.

13. Loveday HP, Wilson JA, Pratt RJ, et al. epic3: national evidence-based guidelines for preventing healthcare-associated infections in NHS hospitals in England. *J Hosp Infect* 2014; **86 Suppl 1**: S1–70.

14. Tenke P, Kovacs B, Bjerklund Johansen TE, et al. European and Asian guidelines on management and prevention of catheter-associated urinary tract infections. *Int J Antimicrob Agents* 2008; **31 Suppl 1**: S68–78.

15. National Health and Medical Research Council. Australian Guidelines for the Prevention and Control of Infection in Healthcare (2019). Canberra: National Health and Medical Research Council; 2019.

16. Centers for Disease Control and Prevention (NHSN). Urinary Tract Infection (Catheter-Associated Urinary Tract Infection [CAUTI] and Non-Catheter-Associated Urinary Tract Infection [UTI]) Events 2020. https://www.cdc.gov/nhsn/PDFs/pscManual/7pscCAUTIcurrent.pdf (accessed 10 February 2020).

17. European Centre for Disease Prevention and Control. Point prevalence survey of healthcare-associated infections and antimicrobial use in European acute care hospitals (Protocol version 5.3). Stockholm: European Centre for Disease Prevention and Control; 2016.

18. Centers for Disease Control and Prevention (NHSN). Identifying Healthcare-associated Infections (HAI) for NHSN Surveillance. 2020. https://www.cdc.gov/nhsn/PDFs/pscManual/2PSC_IdentifyingHAIs_NHSNcurrent.pdf (accessed 10 February 2020).

19. Independent Hospital Pricing Authority. Healthcare-associated infections Hospital-acquired complication (HAI HAC) data. In: Independent Hospital Pricing Authority, editor. Sydney, Australia: Independent Hospital Pricing Authority; 2020.

20. Aubron C, Flint AW, Bailey M, et al. Is platelet transfusion associated with hospital-acquired infections in critically ill patients? *Crit Care* 2017; **21**(1): 2.

21. Roth H, Millar JL, Cheng AC, et al. The state of TRUS biopsy sepsis: readmissions to Victorian hospitals with TRUS biopsy-related infection over 5 years. *BJU Int* 2015; **116 Suppl 3**: 49–53.

22. Jarratt LS, Miller ER. The relationship between patient characteristics and the development of a multi-resistant healthcare-associated infection in a private South Australian hospital. *Healthc Inf* 2013; **18**(3): 94–101.

23. Goodes LM, King GK, Rea A, et al. Early urinary tract infection after spinal cord injury: a retrospective inpatient cohort study. *Spinal Cord* 2020; **58**(1): 25–34.

24. Marshall C, Maglinao K. Is it reasonable to apply ICD-10 coding diagnoses to identify healthcare-associated urinary tract infections? *Infect Dis Health* 2018; **23**: S16.

25. Mitchell BG, Ferguson JK. The use of clinical coding data for the surveillance of healthcare-associated urinary tract infections in Australia. *Infect Dis Health* 2016; **21**(1): 32–5.

CHAPTER 4

Pneumonia

Contents

Introduction

Point prevalence studies (PPS) in Australia, Europe and the United States highlight the type and proportion of different healthcare-associated infections (HAIs), with healthcare–associated pneumonia being one of the most frequent HAIs.[1–3] In PPS, approximately 35% of healthcare-associated pneumonia is classified as ventilator–associated

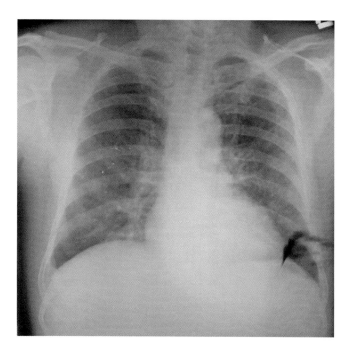

pneumonia (VAP), while the remainder (65%) is considered non-ventilator-associated hospital-acquired pneumonia (NV-HAP).[1] The burden of pneumonia is considerable, with data suggesting that 19% of patients with NV-HAP required transfer into the intensive care unit,[4] which is associated with a prolonged hospital stay and increased patient morbidity and mortality.[5]

There are a number of publications and proposed bundles to prevent VAP. Prevention strategies for VAP include: not implementing ventilatory circuit changes unless specifically indicated, use of a closed endotracheal suction system, strict hand hygiene, incorporation of sedation vacation, weaning protocols into patient care and the use of oral antiseptics.[6-9] In contrast to VAP, the volume of high-quality evidence to support NV-HAP prevention strategies is limited.[10,11] Strategies to prevent NV-HAP include improving oral care in hospitalised patients,[12,13] dysphagia detection and management,[14,15] and increasing movement while in hospital.[16,17] Understanding the burden of healthcare-associated pneumonia may help plan and prioritise prevention strategies.

Definitions and context

There are various definitions of a healthcare-associated pneumonia, including ventilator-associated pneumonia. Examples of these definitions are provided in Table 4.1. For further and more detailed explanations and their applications, please refer to the source document referenced.

Table 4.1 Examples of pneumonia surveillance definitions

Country/ organisation	Subcategory	Overview of definition
Australia		No nationally agreed or defined surveillance definition.
ECDC point prevalence[18] definition★†		Two or more serial chest x-rays or CT scans with a suggestive image of pneumonia for patients with underlying cardiac or pulmonary disease (in patients without underlying cardiac or pulmonary disease, one definitive chest x-ray or CT scan is sufficient) and at least one of the following: • fever > 38°C with no other cause • leucopenia (< 4000 WBC/mm^3) or leucocytosis ≥ 12,000 WBC/mm^3

Table 4.1 Examples of pneumonia surveillance definitions—cont'd

Country/ organisation	Subcategory	Overview of definition

		and at least one of the following (or at least two if clinical pneumonia only = PN 4 and PN 5):
		• new onset of purulent sputum or change in character of sputum (colour, odour, quantity, consistency)
		• cough or dyspnoea or tachypnoea
		• suggestive auscultation (rales or bronchial breath sounds), rhonchi, wheezing
		• worsening gas exchange (e.g. O_2 desaturation or increased oxygen requirements or increased ventilation demand)
		and according to the used diagnostic method:
		a. bacteriologic diagnostic test performed by:
		  • positive quantitative culture from minimally contaminated lower respiratory tract specimen (PN 1)
		  • positive quantitative culture from possibly contaminated LRT specimen (PN 2):
		b. alternative microbiology methods (PN 3)
		c. others:
		  • positive sputum culture or non-quantitative LRT specimen culture (PN 4)
		  • no positive microbiology (PN 5).

United States CDC NHSN[19†‡]	Pneumonia (PNEU)	PNEU is identified by using a combination of imaging, clinical and laboratory criteria. The NHSN have several pages detailing the various criteria that may be used for meeting the surveillance definition of healthcare-associated pneumonia.
	Ventilator-associated pneumonia (VAP)	VAP is where the patient is on mechanical ventilation for > 2 calendar days on the date of event, with day of ventilator placement being day 1[‡], AND the ventilator was in place on the date of event or the day before.

*Also required to meet the definition of healthcare-associated. Day 3 onwards; OR day 1 or day 2 AND patient discharged from acute care hospital in preceding 48 hours; OR day 1 or day 2 AND patient has relevant device inserted on this admission prior to onset.
†Abbreviated version, refer to source document for full details.
‡Also meets definition of HAI using the defined window periods.[20]
Note: CDC = Centers for Disease Control. ECDC = European Centre for Disease Prevention and Control. LRT = lower respiratory tract. NHSN = National Healthcare Safety Network. PN = Pneumonia classification. WBC = white blood cells.

This report presents a collation and analysis of the two types of Australian healthcare-associated pneumonia infection data: 1. proportions of pneumonia hospital-acquired complication (HAC) for the period 1 July 2017 to 30 June 2019; and 2. peer-reviewed literature data for the period 1 January 2010 to 31 August 2019. Each of these potential data sources was interrogated to gain insight into the incidence of healthcare-associated pneumonia in Australia and the findings are presented below. There are no publicly available jurisdictional data on healthcare-associated pneumonia.

Findings

1. Healthcare-associated infection due to hospital-acquired complication (HAI HAC) data

Data on HAI HACs in Australia are collected by the Independent Hospital Pricing Authority (IHPA) but are not currently reported or publicly available. These data were provided upon request. The jurisdictions did not grant permission to publish the raw data but gave permission to report data by proportions. The number of HAI HAC pneumonia are thus presented as a proportion. The raw data from which these proportions were calculated were provided by the IHPA.[21]

The burden of pneumonia in Australian public hospitals in proportions, as identified by HAI HAC data, by state and territory for 2017–2018 and 2018–2019 is presented in Table 4.2 and Figure 4.1. Over both time periods, 87% of reported pneumonias

Table 4.2 Nationwide distribution of HAC HAI pneumonia by jurisdiction (%)

Jurisdiction	Timeframe	
	1 July 2017 – 30 June 2018	1 July 2018 – 30 June 2019
NSW	28.2	28.2
Vic.	29.6	32.7
Qld	17.2	16.0
SA	12.1	10.2
WA	6.8	6.4
Tas.	2.9	3.1
NT	1.1	1.3
ACT	2.1	2.1

Note: ACT = Australian Capital Territory. NSW = New South Wales. NT = Northern Territory. Qld = Queensland. SA = South Australia. Tas. = Tasmania. Vic. = Victoria. WA = Western Australia.
(Source: Compiled from IHPA data.)

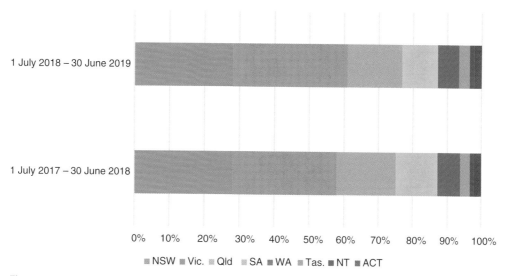

Figure 4.1 *Nationwide distribution of HAC HAI pneumonia by jurisdiction (%)*
Note: ACT = Australian Capital Territory. NSW = New South Wales. NT = Northern Territory. Qld = Queensland. SA = South Australia. Tas. = Tasmania. Vic. = Victoria. WA = Western Australia.
(Source: Compiled from IHPA data.)

occurred in New South Wales, Victoria, Queensland and South Australia. Proportions of pneumonias (%) in each jurisdiction were generally consistent across the time periods.

2. Jurisdictional healthcare-associated infection data

No data from jurisdictions on the surveillance on pneumonia was identified.

3. Peer-reviewed literature data

Table 4.3 summarises the findings from articles identified from the peer-reviewed literature. Studies were conducted in New South Wales,[22] South Australia[23] and Western Australia[24] and two studies were conducted in several jurisdictions.[2,25] There was heterogeneity of the studies with respect to population groups, design, outcome measures and definitions used (see Table 4.5). For these reasons, pooling of data was not possible. Other relevant literature is listed in Table 4.4. The highest reported incidence of pneumonia was 12.4% in a post-cardiac surgery population.[25] The point prevalence of pneumonia was found to be 2.4% in a study involving 19 Australian hospitals.[2]

Table 4.3 Data on pneumonia identified from literature research

Lead author	Year	Location (no. of hospitals)	Year(s) study was undertaken	Population	Type of HAI monitored	Key finding
Gautam[22]	2012	NSW (1)	2010–2011	PICU	VAP	7.02/1000 ventilation days 18 VAP episodes in 269 patients (6.7%)
Jarratt[23]	2013	SA (1)	2003–2011	All hospital	Pneumonia	2.9% MRO pneumonia (3/103) 2.1% non-MRO pneumonia (19/914)
Kelly[24]	2017	WA (1)	2000–2002, 2010–2012	184 patients who underwent major lower limb amputation	Pneumonia	6.9% (6/87) years 2000–2002 3.1% (3/97) years 2010–2012
Russo[2]	2019	All except NT (19)	2018	2767 acute adult inpatients	Pneumonia	2.4% point prevalence (67/2767) (95% CI: 1.9–3.1)
Sanagou[25]	2016	Not specified (16)	2001–2011	Post-cardiac surgical pneumonia	Pneumonia	5.1% (2,229/43,691) Range 0.7–12.4% across hospitals

Note: MRO = multi-resistant organism. NSW = New South Wales. NT = Northern Territory. PICU = paediatric intensive care unit. SA = South Australia. VAP = ventilator-associated pneumonia. WA = Western Australia.

Table 4.4 Other related data identified from literature research

Lead author	Year	Location (no. of hospitals)	Year(s) study was undertaken	Population	Type of HAI monitored	Key finding
Brogan[26]	2014	Australian tertiary hospitals (6)	2010	All hospitals: stroke patients	Respiratory infection	17%
Jarratt[23]	2013	SA (1)	2003–2011	All hospital	Chest infection	MRO: 0; non-MRO: 9 (1%)
Macesic[27]	2013	2010: all Australian jurisdictions; 2011: Vic., ACT, SA, WA (23)	2010 and 2011	All hospital	Nosocomial influenza	26 (4.3%) of the 598 confirmed diagnoses of influenza nosocomial
Parkash[28]	2019	ACT (1)	2017	292 hospitalised adults who tested positive for influenza via real-time PCR testing from any respiratory sample	Influenza	9.6% of influenza diagnoses HCA (28 of 292); 0.17 HCA influenza cases by 100 admissions (28/16,112 admissions)
Sanagou[25]	2016	Not specified (16)	2001–2011	All hospital	Chest infection	MRO: 0; non-MRO: 9 (1%)

Note: ACT = Australian Capital Territory. MRO = multi-resistant organism. PCR = polymerase chain reaction. SA = South Australia. VAP = ventilator-associated pneumonia. Vic. = Victoria. WA = Western Australia.

Synthesis and summary

Despite pneumonia being one of the most common HAIs acquired in hospital, at the time of data collection, no Australian state or territory currently had publicly available data on the frequency of pneumonia. The distribution of the burden of pneumonia HAC data across the country, as presented in Table 4.1 and Figure 4.1, potentially reflects hospital activity and/or population. However, as we were unable to publish numerator or denominator data for HAC data, interpretation of these data is not possible.

Table 4.5 HAI definitions used in the identified studies

Lead author	Year	HAI definition used
Brogan[26]	2014	Unknown
Gautam[22]	2012	Ventilator-associated pneumonia (VAP) refers to pneumonia that develops in patients on invasive mechanical ventilation
Jarratt[23]	2013	Defined as any localised or systemic condition resulting from an infectious agent or toxin for which no evidence was apparent on admission to the acute care setting
Kelly[24]	2017	ICD-10 coding data
Macesic[27]	2013	Nosocomial influenza: PCR-confirmed influenza where the onset of symptoms was more than 2 days after the patient's admission or, if this was not known, where the date of the positive test was more than 7 days after admission
Parkash[28]	2019	HA influenza: symptom onset more than 48 hours after admission to study hospital for non-respiratory-illness-related reason; if symptom onset unknown, lab diagnosis of influenza ≥ 7 days after admission was defined as a hospital-acquired case.
Russo[2]	2019	ECDC point prevalence definition
Sanagou[25]	2016	Pneumonia diagnosed by one of the following: positive non-quantitative cultures of sputum or trans-tracheal aspirate with a recognised pathogen and clinical and radiological features consistent with pneumonia with onset after surgery

Note: ECDC = European Centre for Disease Prevention and Control. HA = hospital-acquired. PCR = polymerase chain reaction.

At this point in time in Australia, the clearest picture of the burden of pneumonia comes from the peer-reviewed literature. However, these data are limited by publication bias, as well as challenges interpreting data from studies that use different approaches, populations and case definitions of pneumonia.

References

1. Magill SS, Edwards JR, Bamberg W, et al. Multistate point-prevalence survey of health care–associated infections. *N Engl J Med* 2014; **370**(13): 1198–208.
2. Russo PL, Stewardson AJ, Cheng AC, et al. The prevalence of healthcare-associated infections among adult inpatients at nineteen large Australian acute-care public hospitals: a point prevalence survey. *Antimicrob Resist Infect Control* 2019; **8**(1): 114.
3. European Centre for Disease Prevention and Control. Point prevalence survey of healthcare-associated infections and antimicrobial use in European acute care hospitals. Stockholm: European Centre for Disease Prevention and Control; 2013.

4. Centers for Medicare & Medicaid Services. Hospital-Acquired Condition Reduction Program Fiscal Year 2019 Fact Sheet. 2019. https://www.cms.gov/Medicare/Medicare-Fee-for-Service-Payment/AcuteInpatientPPS/Downloads/HAC-Reduction-Program-Fact-Sheet.pdf (accessed 12 February 2019).

5. Magill SS, O'Leary E, Janelle SJ, et al. Changes in Prevalence of Health Care–Associated Infections in US Hospitals. *N Engl J Med* 2018; **379**(18): 1732–44.

6. Labeau SO, Van de Vyver K, Brusselaers N, et al. Prevention of ventilator-associated pneumonia with oral antiseptics: a systematic review and meta-analysis. *Lancet Infect Dis* 2011; **11**(11): 845–54.

7. Rello J, Lode H, Cornaglia G, et al. A European care bundle for prevention of ventilator-associated pneumonia. *Intensive Care Med* 2010; **36**(5): 773–80.

8. Dodek P, Keenan S, Cook D, et al. Evidence-based clinical practice guideline for the prevention of ventilator-associated pneumonia. *Ann Intern Med* 2004; **141**(4): 305–13.

9. Rello J, Afonso E, Lisboa T, et al. A care bundle approach for prevention of ventilator-associated pneumonia. *Clin Microbiol Infect* 2013; **19**(4): 363–9.

10. Mitchell BG, Russo PL, Cheng AC, et al. Strategies to reduce non-ventilator-associated hospital-acquired pneumonia: A systematic review. *Infect Dis Health* 2019; **24**(4): 229–39.

11. Passaro L, Harbarth S, Landelle C. Prevention of hospital-acquired pneumonia in non-ventilated adult patients: a narrative review. *Antimicrob Resist Infect Control* 2016; **5**: 43.

12. Bellissimo-Rodrigues WT, Menegueti MG, Gaspar GG, et al. Effectiveness of a dental care intervention in the prevention of lower respiratory tract nosocomial infections among intensive care patients: a randomized clinical trial. *Infect Control Hosp Epidemiol* 2014; **35**(11): 1342–8.

13. Bourigault C, Lietard C, Golmard JL, et al. Impact of bucco-dental healthcare on the prevention of pneumonia in geriatrics: a cluster-randomised trial. *J Hosp Infect* 2011; **77**(1): 78–80.

14. Schrock JW, Lou L, Ball BAW, et al. The use of an emergency department dysphagia screen is associated with decreased pneumonia in acute strokes. *Am J Emerg Med* 2018; **36**(12): 2152–4.

15. Titsworth WL, Abram J, Fullerton A, et al. Prospective quality initiative to maximize dysphagia screening reduces hospital-acquired pneumonia prevalence in patients with stroke. *Stroke* 2013; **44**(11): 3154–60.

16. Boden I, Skinner EH, Browning L, et al. Preoperative physiotherapy for the prevention of respiratory complications after upper abdominal surgery: pragmatic, double blinded, multicentre randomised controlled trial. *BMJ* 2018; **360**: j5916.

17. Cuesy PG, Sotomayor PL, Pina JO. Reduction in the incidence of poststroke nosocomial pneumonia by using the 'turn-mob' program. *J Stroke Cerebrovasc Dis* 2010; **19**(1): 23–8.

18. European Centre for Disease Prevention and Control. Point prevalence survey of healthcare-associated infections and antimicrobial use in European acute care hospitals (Protocol version 5.3). Stockholm: European Centre for Disease Prevention and Control; 2016.

19. Centers for Disease Control and Prevention (NHSN). Pneumonia (Ventilator-associated [VAP] and non-ventilator-associated Pneumonia [PNEU]) Event 2020. https://www.cdc.gov/nhsn/pdfs/pscmanual/6pscvapcurrent.pdf (accessed 10 February 2020).

20. Centers for Disease Control and Prevention (NHSN). Identifying Healthcare-associated Infections (HAI) for NHSN Surveillance. 2020. https://www.cdc.gov/nhsn/PDFs/pscManual/2PSC_IdentifyingHAIs_NHSNcurrent.pdf (accessed 10 February 2020).

21. Independent Hospital Pricing Authority. Healthcare-associated infections Hospital-acquired complication (HAI HAC) data. In: Independent Hospital Pricing Authority, editor. Sydney, Australia: Independent Hospital Pricing Authority; 2020.

22. Gautam A, Ganu SS, Tegg OJ, et al. Ventilator-associated pneumonia in a tertiary paediatric intensive care unit: a 1-year prospective observational study. *Crit Care Resusc* 2012; **14**(4): 283–9.

23. Jarratt LS, Miller ER. The relationship between patient characteristics and the development of a multi-resistant healthcare-associated infection in a private South Australian hospital. *Healthc Inf* 2013; **18**(3): 94–101.

24. Kelly DA, Pedersen S, Tosenovsky P, et al. Major Lower Limb Amputation: Outcomes are Improving. *Ann Vasc Surg* 2017; **45**: 29–34.

25. Sanagou M, Leder K, Cheng A, et al. Associations of hospital characteristics with nosocomial pneumonia after cardiac surgery can impact on standardized infection rates. *Epidemiol Infect* 2016; **144**(5): 1065–74.
26. Brogan E, Langdon C, Brookes K, et al. Respiratory infections in acute stroke: nasogastric tubes and immobility are stronger predictors than dysphagia. *Dysphagia* 2014; **29**(3): 340–5.
27. Macesic N, Kotsimbos TC, Kelly P, et al. Hospital-acquired influenza in an Australian sentinel surveillance system. *Med J Aust* 2013; **198**(7): 370–2.
28. Parkash N, Beckingham W, Andersson P, et al. Hospital-acquired influenza in an Australian tertiary Centre 2017: a surveillance-based study. *BMC Pulm Med* 2019; **19**(1): 79.

CHAPTER 5

Bloodstream infection

Contents

Introduction

Bloodstream infections (BSIs) cause significant morbidity and mortality.[1,2] A recent review of data collected over a 4-year period from the European Centre for Disease Prevention and Control (ECDC) identified that 3.5% of intensive care unit patients acquired a BSI, with an estimated attributable mortality of 5.0% (95% CI: 3.9–6.2) and an attributable excess length of intensive care unit (ICU) stay of 14 days.[3]

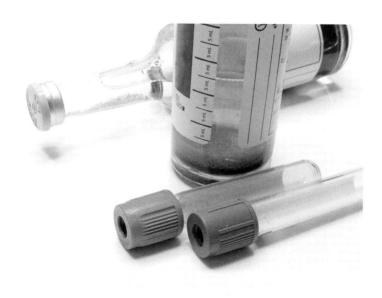

International point prevalence studies have identified that of all healthcare-associated infections (HAIs), the frequency of BSI ranges from 8.7% to 10.6%.[4-7] A recent Australian national point prevalence study conducted in 19 large acute care hospitals identified that 10.0% of HAIs identified were BSIs.[8]

Staphylococcus aureus bacteraemia (SAB) is a key performance indicator for all acute care hospitals in Australia under the Australian Health Performance Network. Episodes of SAB are commonly associated with medical procedures and potentially preventable, thus they are generally considered an indicator of quality of care.[9] Given this, SAB data is collated annually and published through the Australian Institute of Health and Welfare's MyHospitals website.[10] Data are risk adjusted according to hospital peer group and case type. Currently, a performance benchmark for public healthcare-associated SAB is set at 2.0 per 10,000 patient days. Data from 2017–2018 identified that all states and territories reported public hospital SAB rates below the national benchmark.[11]

Definitions and context

Examples of BSI surveillance definitions are provided in Table 5.1. Both ECDC and the United States Centers for Disease Control and Prevention (CDC) definitions include laboratory confirmation and other clinical elements depending on the organism identified. Once established as a BSI, further criteria can be worked through to determine a source (not included in Table 5.1). The Australian definition of SAB commences with a positive blood culture for *S. aureus*, and then other criteria are sought to determine if it is considered healthcare associated. For further and more detailed explanations and their applications, please refer to the source document referenced.

The report presents a collation and analysis of the three types of Australian healthcare-associated bloodstream infection data: 1. proportions of bloodstream infection hospital-acquired complication (HAC) for the period 1 July 2017 to 30 June 2019; 2. publicly available state and territory jurisdiction surveillance data for the period 1 July 2017 to 30 June 2019; and 3. peer-reviewed literature data for the period 1 January 2010 to 31 August 2019. Each of these potential data sources was interrogated to gain insight into the incidence of healthcare-associated bloodstream infection in Australia and the findings are presented on the following pages.

Findings

1. Healthcare-associated infection due to hospital-acquired complication (HAI HAC) data

Data on HAI HACs in Australia are collected by the Independent Hospital Pricing Authority (IHPA) but are not currently reported or publicly available. These data

Table 5.1 Example definitions

Country/ organisation	Subcategory	Overview of definition
Australia[12]	SAB	A patient episode of *Staphylococcus aureus* bacteraemia (SAB) is a positive blood culture for *Staphylococcus aureus*. For surveillance purposes, only the first isolate per patient is counted, unless at least 14 days has passed without a positive culture, after which an additional episode is recorded. A SAB will be considered to be a healthcare-associated event if: EITHER CRITERION A The patient's first SAB positive blood culture was collected more than 48 hours after hospital admission or less than 48 hours after discharge. OR CRITERION B The patient's first positive SAB blood culture was collected less than or equal to 48 hours after hospital admission and one or more of the following key clinical criteria was met for the patient episode of SAB: 1. SAB is a complication of the presence of an indwelling medical device (e.g. intravascular line, haemodialysis vascular access, CSF shunt, urinary catheter) 2. SAB occurs within 30 days of a surgical procedure where the SAB is related to the surgical site 3. SAB was diagnosed within 48 hours of a related invasive instrumentation or incision 4. SAB is associated with neutropenia★ contributed to by cytotoxic therapy.
United States CDC NHSN[13]		Primary bloodstream infection (BSI): a laboratory confirmed bloodstream infection (LCBI) that is not secondary to an infection at another body site.

Continued

Table 5.1 Example definitions—cont'd

Country/ organisation	Subcategory	Overview of definition

Europe (ECDC)[14]	BSI: Bloodstream infection BSI: Laboratory-confirmed bloodstream infection	• One positive blood culture for a recognised pathogen OR
		• patient has at least one of the following signs or symptoms: fever (> 38°C), chills or hypotension AND
		• two positive blood cultures for a common skin contaminant (from two separate blood samples, usually within 48 hours).
		Skin contaminants = coagulase-negative staphylococci, *Micrococcus* sp., *Propionibacterium acnes*, *Bacillus* sp., *Corynebacterium* sp.
		Note: This definition corresponds to the former HELICS BSI-A definition; BSI-B (single blood culture for skin contaminants in patients with central vascular catheter and adapted treatment) was deleted following recommendations at an ECDC expert meeting in January 2009 and subsequent confirmation at the annual meeting.
		Sources of bloodstream infection:
		• Catheter-related: the same microorganism was cultured from the catheter or symptoms improve within 48 hours after removal of the catheter (C-PVC: peripheral catheter, C-CVC: central vascular catheter). Important: Report C-CVC or C-PVC BSI as CRI3-CVC or CRI3-PVC respectively if microbiologically confirmed; see CRI3 definition.
		• Secondary to another infection: the same microorganism was isolated from another infection site, or strong clinical evidence exists that bloodstream infection was secondary to another infection site, invasive diagnostic procedure or foreign body:
		   ○ pulmonary (S-PUL);
		   ○ urinary tract infection (S-UTI);
		   ○ digestive tract infection (S-DIG);
		   ○ surgical site infection (S-SSI);
		   ○ skin and soft tissue (S-SST);
		   ○ other (S-OTH).
		• Unknown origin (UO): none of the above, bloodstream infection of unknown origin (verified during survey and no source found).
		• Unknown (UNK): no information available about the source of the bloodstream infection or information missing.

Table 5.1 Example definitions—cont'd

Country/organisation	Subcategory	Overview of definition
		Note: Primary bloodstream infections include catheter-related BSI and BSI of unknown origin. A CVC-associated bloodstream infection in accordance with CDC NHSN definitions (as opposed to CVC-related BSI) is a primary BSI with central venous catheter use (even intermittent) in the 48 hours preceding the onset of the infection: therefore, the presence of 'the relevant device' (central/peripheral vascular catheter) in the 48 hours before onset of infection is collected even in the absence of microbiological confirmation.

Table 5.2 Nationwide distribution of HAC HAI BSIs by jurisdiction (%)

Jurisdiction	Timeframe	
	1 July 2017 – 30 June 2018	*1 July 2018 – 30 June 2019*
NSW	23.8	22.8
Vic.	39.6	44.4
Qld	19.9	18.4
SA	5.2	3.8
WA	6.6	5.9
Tas.	1.9	2.0
NT	1.2	0.9
ACT	1.8	1.9

Note: ACT = Australian Capital Territory. NSW = New South Wales. NT = Northern Territory. Qld = Queensland. SA = South Australia. Tas. = Tasmania. Vic. = Victoria. WA = Western Australia.
(Source: Compiled from IHPA data.)

were provided upon request. The jurisdictions did not grant permission to publish the raw data but gave permission to report data by proportions. The number of HAI HAC BSIs are thus presented as a proportion. The raw data from which these proportions were calculated were provided by the IHPA.[15]

The burden of bloodstream infections in Australian public hospitals, as identified by HAI HAC data, by state and territory for 2017–2018 and 2018–2019 is presented in Table 5.2 and Figure 5.1. Over both time periods, 83% to 85% of reported BSIs occurred in New South Wales, Victoria and Queensland (the most populous states)

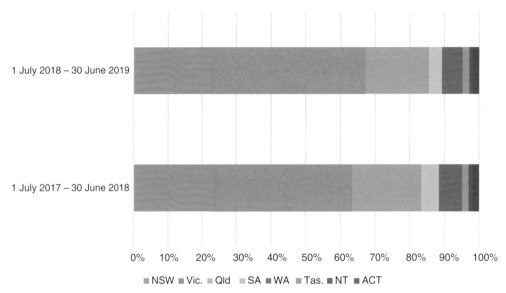

Figure 5.1 *Nationwide distribution of HAC HAI Bloodstream Infections by jurisdiction (%)*
Note: ACT = Australian Capital Territory. NSW = New South Wales. NT = Northern Territory. Qld = Queensland.
SA = South Australia. Tas. = Tasmania. Vic. = Victoria. WA = Western Australia.
(Source: Compiled from IHPA data.)

over both time periods. In 2018–2019, reported BSIs in Victoria increased by almost 5%. Proportions of BSIs (%) in the other jurisdictions remained stable.

2. Jurisdictional HAI data

BSI data from Australian jurisdictions is identified in Table 5.3.

3. Peer-reviewed literature data

Table 5.4 summarises the findings from articles identified from the peer-reviewed literature. Eighteen studies were identified, at least one study from each jurisdiction. There was heterogeneity in the type of BSI monitored, population groups and the definitions used (Table 5.5).

Synthesis and summary

Despite the relatively simple and uniform international definitions of a BSI, *Staphylococcus aureus* bacteraemia is the only nationally reported HAI in Australia. Data is risk adjusted, reported annually and used as a performance indicator.

HAC data are administrative data collected by hospitals originally designed for accounting purposes. Multiple studies have demonstrated their unreliability in identifying

Table 5.3 BSI data by Australian jurisdiction

Year	ACT	NSW	NT	Qld	SA[16]	Tas.[17]	Vic.[18]	WA[19]
2017–2018	–	–	–	–	SAB n = 0.83/10,000 OBD Total HA BSI 2017 n = 688	SAB = 1.0/10,000 OBD	SAB = 0.67/10,000 OBD	SAB = 0.7/10,000 OBD Haemodialysis access-associated BSI: AVF = 0.07 per patient (95% CI: 0.03–0.14) AVG = 0.26 per patient (95% CI: 0.69–1.38)
2018–2019[11]	SAB 0.82	SAB 0.73	SAB 0.47	SAB 0.76	SAB 0.61	SAB 0.83	SAB 0.77	SAB 0.86

Note: – indicates that data was not available. ACT = Australian Capital Territory. NSW = New South Wales. NT = Northern Territory. OBD = occupied bed days. SAB = *Staphylococcus aureus* bacteraemia. Qld = Queensland. SA = South Australia. Tas. = Tasmania. Vic. = Victoria. WA = Western Australia.

HAI.[38] As well as unreliability, the HAC data provided here are unable to be interpreted given the lack of both numerator and denominator data. The data provided indicate that more HAI HAC BSIs are reported from the bigger states, which is to be expected given there are more hospitals in the larger states.

Four states publicly reported SAB data in 2017/18, while data from each state and territory is available for 2018–2019 from reports generated by the Australian Institute of Health and Welfare. Of the four states that reported data for 2017–2018, two demonstrated a reduction in SAB in data reported for 2018–2019. For the 2018–2019 period, the rate of SAB by jurisdiction ranged from 0.47 to 0.86 per 10,000 patient days.

Eighteen peer-reviewed studies were identified. Of these only one was a national study,[28] another multistate[32] and all others were single state studies. Six of the single state studies were conducted in New South Wales, four in Victoria and three in Queensland. Six of the studies included all hospital patients in the study population, while four derived data from intensive care unit populations.

Due to the heterogeneity of the studies, it is not possible to combine or compare data for analysis. Definitions as listed in Table 5.5 vary enormously, and outcome data is expressed as a rate per unit beds or patient bed days, or a proportion of patients with a BSI.

Table 5.4 Data on BSIs identified from literature research

Lead author	Year	Location (no. of hospitals)	Year(s) study was undertaken	Population	Type of HAI monitored	Key finding
Alcorn[20]	2013	Qld (1)	2001–2011	All hospital	GN BSI	181 non-inpatient GN BSI (of 841 HA BSI) 259 inpatient GN BSI (of 841 HA BSI)
					GP BSI	149 non-inpatient GP BSI (of 841 HA BSI) 252 inpatient GP BSI (of 841 HA BSI)
Aminzadeh[21]	2019	Vic. (1)	2016–2018	All patients diagnosed with CVC–BSI in non-ICU settings of hospital	CVC-BSIs	23 cases or 1.2/10,000 bed days
Anderson[22]	2015	NSW (1)	2009–2013	All patients who presented to hospital with sepsis following TRUS biopsy	Bacteraemia following TRUS biopsy	Average rate of 1.5% bacteraemia over 5 years
Aubron[23]	2017	Vic. (2)	2008–2013	ICU patients (PLT recipients versus non-PLT recipients)	Bacteraemia	All patients: 178/18,965 (0.9%); PLT recipients: 99/2250 (4.4%); non-PLT recipients: 79/16,715 (0.5%)

Aubron[24]	2015	Vic. (1)	2006–2011	ICU	BSI associated with positive urine cultures: candiduria/bacteriuria; bacteriuria/candiduria episodes	0.17 positive urine culture–associated BSI/1000 ICU days/6.4 ICU-acquired positive urine cultures/1000 ICU days; 6 patients had this association
Austin[25]	2017	NSW (1)	2011–2014	98 ECMO patients	Bloodstream	8.8 per 1000 ECMO days
Betts[26]	2019	Qld (?)	2009–2015	All inpatient live births in Qld in study period	Sepsis	0.54%
Campbell[27]	2019	WA (1)	2014–2015	11,774 processed blood culture bottles from PICU	BSI SAB	207 BSIs, of which 122 (58.9%) were HCA 10 (8.2%) cases were SAB
Coombs[28]	2013	NSW, Vic., Qld, NT, ACT, Tas., WA, SA (29)	2011	All hospital	Staphylococcus aureus isolates Site of Staphylococcus aureus isolates Methicillin-resistant Staphylococcus aureus	NSW/ACT: 639; Qld/NT: 591; SA: 254; Vic./Tas.: 541; WA: 332 Skin and soft tissue: 1661 (95% CI: 68.6–72.3); respiratory: 404 (95% CI: 15.6–18.7); blood: 153 (95% CI: 5.5–7.6); urine: 88 (95% CI: 3.0–4.6); sterile body cavity: 49 (95% CI: 1.5–2.7); cerebrospinal fluid (95% CI: 0.01–0.3) NSW/ACT: 253/639 (95% CI: 33.1–40.6); Qld/NT: 180/591 (95% CI: 26.9–34.3; SA: 55/254 (95% CI: 17.0–27.1); Vic./Tas.: 177/541 (95% CI: 28.9–36.8); WA: 66/332 (95% CI: 15.9–24.5)

Continued

Table 5.4 Data on BSIs identified from literature research—cont'd

Lead author	Year	Location (no. of hospitals)	Year(s) study was undertaken	Population	Type of HAI monitored	Key finding
Ezzatzadegan[29]	2012	NSW (1)	2000–2010	Renal transplantation centre	Invasive fungal infection	10/471 patients (2.1%, 95% CI: 0.7%–3.4%)
Jarratt[30]	2013	SA (1)	2003–2011	All hospital	BSI	MRO: 2 (1.9%); non-MRO: 105 (11.5%)
Mathot[31]	2015	Vic. (1)	2002–2012	PICU	Gram-positive bacteria Gram-negative bacteria Fungi	533 (36%, 445 patients); 1480 new infections 760 (51.4%, 561 patients) 187 (12.6%, 169 patients)
Mitchell[32]	2014	WA, ACT, Tas., SA (132)	2002–2013	All hospital	Staphylococcus aureus bacteraemia MSSA MRSA	Aggregate incidence 0.90/10,000 patient days (95% CI: 0.86–0.93); 2733 HOB cases 0.62/10,000 patient days (95% CI: 0.60–0.65) 0.28/10,000 patient days (95% CI: 0.26–0.29)
Mumford[33]	2014	NSW (77)	2009–2012	All hospital	Staphylococcus aureus bacteraemia	0.77/10,000 bed days (2012)
Munro[34]	2018	WA (1)	2011–2013	Prospectively identified SAB patients	Staphylococcus aureus bacteraemia (healthcare-associated)	12 healthcare-associated SAB cases. HCA SAB 0.38/10,000 bed days (24.5% of combined SAB rate of 1.57/10,000)

Ou[35]	2017	NSW (82)	2007–2012	144,503 adult elective surgical patients admitted to 82 public acute hospitals	Sepsis	1.30%
Roediger[36]	2017	NSW (1)	2006–2011	174 clinical episodes of SAB	*Staphylococcus aureus* bacteraemia	Rate of HCA SBA over 5-year study period: 0.6/1000 admissions
Si[37]	2016	Qld (23)	2008–2012	All hospital	HA BSI	5.97/10,000 patient days (95% CI: 5.83–6.12); 6410 cases
					HA IVC-BSI	1.85/10,000 patient days (95% CI: 1.77–1.93); 1983 cases
					HA *Staphylococcus aureus* BSI	1.01/10,000 patient days (95% CI: 0.95–1.07); 1085 cases
					HA MRSA BSI	0.26/10,000 patient days (95% CI: 0.23–0.29); 281 cases

Note: ACT = Australian Capital Territory. BSI = bloodstream infection. CVC = central venous catheter. ECMO = extracorporeal membrane oxygenation. GN = gram-negative. GP = gram-positive. HA = hospital-acquired. HOB = hospital-onset bacteraemia. ICU = intensive care unit. IVC = intravascular catheter. MRO = multi-resistant organism. MRSA = methicillin-resistant *Staphylococcus aureus*. MSSA = methicillin-susceptible *Staphylococcus aureus*. NSW = New South Wales. NT = Northern Territory. PICU = paediatric intensive care unit. PLT = platelet. Qld = Queensland. SA = South Australia. SAB = *Staphylococcus aureus* bacteraemia. Tas. = Tasmania. Vic. = Victoria. WA = Western Australia.

Table 5.5 HAI definitions used in the identified studies

Lead author	Year	HAI definition used
Alcorn[20]	2013	Australian Council for Safety and Quality in Health Care Definition
Aminzadeh[21]	2019	CVC-BSIs according to NHSN definition within the 18-month research period. BSI status laboratory-confirmed via 'CVC-BSI' = BSI occurs during presence of CVC, or within 48 hours of CVC removal
Anderson[22]	2015	A case was defined as a patient who presented to hospital with sepsis due to suspected or confirmed infection related to the genitourinary tract or where no other focus of infection was clinically evident within 14 days of undergoing a TRUS biopsy from 2009 until 2013; sepsis was defined according to the ACCP/SCCM (1991) criteria as a systemic inflammatory response syndrome in the presence of an infective process
Aubron[23]	2017	'Infection' = bacteraemia or bacteriuria occurring in ICU after 48 hours of ICU stay
Aubron[24]	2015	UTI: NHSN definition
Austin[25]	2017	BSI: definition modified from CDC NHSN; considered ECMO-related if positive cultures collected at least 48 hours after ECMO commencement and within 24 hours of ECMO cessation
Betts[26]	2019	ICD-10-AM code puerperal sepsis
Campbell[27]	2019	Health Infection Surveillance Western Australia definitions that concur with the CSC NHSN definitions used to determine community-acquired bacteraemia (CAB), healthcare-associated *Staphylococcus aureus* bacteraemia (HASAB), CLABSI and bacteraemia secondary to mucosal barrier injury (MBI); definition for healthcare-associated bacteraemia (HA-B) from NHSN CDC HA-SAB definition as there is no recognised standard definition
Coombs[28]	2013	*S. aureus* isolates from hospital inpatients (hospital stay > 48 hours at the time of specimen collection)
Ezzatzadegan[29]	2012	Positive culture
Jarratt[30]	2013	HAI defined using CDC definitions (2012)
Mathot[31]	2015	Infections identified by positive bacterial or fungal culture from blood and/or bronchoalveolar lavage
Mitchell[32]	2014	HO-SAB, which was defined as 1 or more blood cultures positive for *S. aureus*, taken from a patient who had been admitted to hospital for > 48 hours; the term 'HO-SAB' is defined as any case of SAB occurring > 48 hours after admission

Table 5.5 HAI definitions used in the identified studies—cont'd

Lead author	Year	HAI definition used
Mumford[33]	2014	*Staphylococcus aureus* bacteraemia where the first positive blood culture is collected > 48 hours after hospital admission or < 48 hours after discharge, or SAB is a complication of the presence of an indwelling medical device; SAB occurs within 30 days of a surgical procedure and is related to the surgical site; an invasive instrumentation or incision related to the SAB was performed within 48 hours; or SAB is associated with neutropenia (< 1 × 109) related to cytotoxic therapy
Munro[34]	2018	*S. aureus* bacteraemia defined by detection of *S. aureus* in blood cultures in the presence of a consistent clinical illness; 'hospital acquired': positive blood culture taken 48 or more hours after admission 'community-onset, healthcare-associated': not hospital-acquired, but there was medical device in situ; 'community-acquired' if didn't meet criteria for either of the other two prior categories

Note: CA = community-acquired. CDC = Centers for Disease Control and Prevention. CLABSI = central line-associated bloodstream infection. CVC = central venous catheter. ECMO = extracorporeal membrane oxygenation. HA = hospital-acquired. HO = hospital-onset. NHSN = National Healthcare Safety Network. SAB = *Staphylococcus aureus* bacteraemia.

References

1. Goudie A, Dynan L, Brady PW, et al. Attributable cost and length of stay for central line-associated bloodstream infections. *Pediatrics* 2014; **133**(6): e1525–32.
2. Maki DG, Kluger DM, Crnich CJ. The risk of bloodstream infection in adults with different intravascular devices: a systematic review of 200 published prospective studies. *Mayo Clin Proc* 2006; **81**(9): 1159–71.
3. European Centre for Disease Prevention and Control. Incidence and attributable mortality of healthcare-associated infections in intensive care units in Europe, 2008–2012. Stockholm: ECDC, 2018.
4. Cai Y, Venkatachalam I, Tee NW, et al. Prevalence of Healthcare-Associated Infections and Antimicrobial Use Among Adult Inpatients in Singapore Acute-Care Hospitals: Results From the First National Point Prevalence Survey. *Clin Infect Dis* 2017; **64**(suppl_2): S61–7.
5. Cairns S, Gibbons C, Milne A, et al. Results from the third Scottish National Prevalence Survey: is a population health approach now needed to prevent healthcare-associated infections? *J Hosp Infect* 2018; **99**(3): 312–7.
6. European Centre for Disease Prevention and Control. Point prevalence survey of healthcare-associated infections and antimicrobial use in European acute care hospitals. Stockholm: European Centre for Disease Prevention and Control; 2013.
7. Magill SS, Edwards JR, Bamberg W, et al. Multistate point-prevalence survey of healthcare-associated infections. *N Engl J Med* 2014; **370**(13): 1198–208.
8. Russo PL, Stewardson AJ, Cheng AC, et al. The prevalence of healthcare-associated infections among adult inpatients at nineteen large Australian acute-care public hospitals: a point prevalence survey. *Antimicrob Resist Infect Control* 2019; **8**: 114.
9. Collignon P, Cruickshank M, Dreimanis D. *Staphylococcus aureus* bloodstream infections: an important indicator for infection control. Chapter 2: Bloodstream infections—an abridged version. *Healthc Inf* 2009; **14**(4): 165–71.

10. Australian Institute of Health and Welfare. MyHospitals. 2020. https://www.aihw.gov.au/myhospitals (accessed 2 April 2020).

11. Australian Institute of Health and Welfare. Bloodstream infections associated with hospital care 2017–18: Australian hospital statistics. Canberra: AIHW, 2019.

12. Australian Commission on Safety and Quality in Health Care. Implementation Guide for Surveillance of *Staphylococcus aureus* Bacteraemia Sydney, Australia: Australian Commission on Safety and Quality in Health Care, 2011.

13. Centers for Disease Control and Prevention. Bloodstream Infection Event (Central Line-Associated Bloodstream Infection and Non-central Line Associated Bloodstream Infection) *Centers for Disease Control and Prevention*; 2020. p. 49.

14. European Centre for Disease Prevention and Control. Point prevalence survey of healthcare-associated infections and antimicrobial use in European acute care hospitals (Protocol version 5.3). Stockholm: European Centre for Disease Prevention and Control; 2016.

15. Independent Hospital Pricing Authority. Healthcare-associated infections Hospital-acquired complication (HAI HAC) data. In: Independent Hospital Pricing Authority, editor. Sydney, Australia: Independent Hospital Pricing Authority; 2020.

16. Cope C. South Australian Healthcare-associated Infection Surveillance Program: Bloodstream Infection Annual Report 2018. In: Infection Control Service CDCB, editor. Adelaide, South Australia: SA Department for Health and Wellbeing; 2019. p. 25.

17. Wilson F, Anderson T, Wells A. *Staphylococcus aureus* bloodstream infection surveillance. Report, 2010 to 2018. In: Tasmania Department of Health, editor. Hobart: Department of Health, Tasmania; 2019. p. 17.

18. Department of Health and Human Services, The University of Melbourne, The Royal Melbourne Hospital, The Peter Doherty Institute for Infection and Immunity. Healthcare-associated infection in Victoria: Surveillance report for 2016–17 and 2017–18. Melbourne, Australia, 2018.

19. Communicable Disease Control Directorate. Healthcare Infection Surveillance Western Australia: Annual Report 2017–18. Perth, Western Australia, 2018.

20. Alcorn K, Gerrard J, Macbeth D, et al. Seasonal variation in healthcare-associated bloodstream infection: increase in the incidence of gram-negative bacteremia in nonhospitalized patients during summer. *Am J Infect Control* 2013; **41**(12): 1205–8.

21. Aminzadeh Z, Simpson P, Athan E. Central venous catheter associated blood stream infections (CVC-BSIs) in the non-intensive care settings: Epidemiology, microbiology and outcomes. *Infect Dis Health* 2019; **24**(4): 222–8.

22. Anderson E, Leahy O, Cheng AC, et al. Risk factors for infection following prostate biopsy—a case control study. *BMC Infect Dis* 2015; **15**: 580.

23. Aubron C, Flint AW, Bailey M, et al. Is platelet transfusion associated with hospital-acquired infections in critically ill patients? *Crit Care* 2017; **21**(1): 2.

24. Aubron C, Suzuki S, Glassford NJ, et al. The epidemiology of bacteriuria and candiduria in critically ill patients. *Epidemiol Infect* 2015; **143**(3): 653–62.

25. Austin DE, Kerr SJ, Al-Soufi S, et al. Nosocomial infections acquired by patients treated with extra-corporeal membrane oxygenation. *Crit Care Resusc* 2017; **19**(Suppl 1): 68–75.

26. Betts KS, Kisely S, Alati R. Predicting common maternal postpartum complications: leveraging health administrative data and machine learning. *BJOG* 2019; **126**(6): 702–9.

27. Campbell AJ, Blyth CC, Hewison CJ, et al. Lessons learned from a hospital-wide review of blood stream infections for paediatric central line-associated blood stream infection prevention. *J Paediatr Child Health* 2019; **55**(6): 690–4.

28. Coombs GW, Nimmo GR, Pearson JC, et al. Australian Group on Antimicrobial Resistance Hospital-onset *Staphylococcus aureus* Surveillance Programme annual report, 2011. *Commun Dis Intell Q Rep* 2013; **37**(3): E210–18.

29. Ezzatzadegan S, Chen S, Chapman JR. Invasive fungal infections after renal transplantation. *Int J Organ Transplant Med* 2012; **3**(1): 18–25.

30. Jarratt LS, Miller ER. The relationship between patient characteristics and the development of a multi-resistant healthcare-associated infection in a private South Australian hospital. *Healthc Inf* 2013; **18**(3): 94–101.

31. Mathot F, Duke T, Daley AJ, et al. Bacteremia and pneumonia in a tertiary PICU: an 11-year study. *Pediatr Crit Care Med* 2015; **16**(2): 104–13.

32. Mitchell BG, Collignon PJ, McCann R, et al. A major reduction in hospital-onset *Staphylococcus aureus* bacteremia in Australia—12 years of progress: an observational study. *Clin Infect Dis* 2014; **59**(7): 969–75.

33. Mumford V, Reeve R, Greenfield D, et al. Is accreditation linked to hospital infection rates? A 4-year, data linkage study of *Staphylococcus aureus* rates and accreditation scores in 77 Australian acute hospitals. *Int J Qual Health Care* 2015; **27**(6): 479–85.

34. Munro APS, Blyth CC, Campbell AJ, et al. Infection characteristics and treatment of *Staphylococcus aureus* bacteraemia at a tertiary children's hospital. *BMC Infect Dis* 2018; **18**(1): 387.

35. Ou L, Chen J, Hillman K, et al. The impact of post-operative sepsis on mortality after hospital discharge among elective surgical patients: a population-based cohort study. *Crit Care* 2017; **21**(1): 34.

36. Roediger JC, Outhred AC, Shadbolt B, et al. Paediatric *Staphylococcus aureus* bacteraemia: A single-centre retrospective cohort. *J Paediatr Child Health* 2017; **53**(2): 180–6.

37. Si D, Runnegar N, Marquess J, et al. Characterising health care-associated bloodstream infections in public hospitals in Queensland, 2008–2012. *Med J Aust* 2016; **204**(7): 276.

38. van Mourik MS, van Duijn PJ, Moons KG, et al. Accuracy of administrative data for surveillance of healthcare-associated infections: a systematic review. *BMJ Open* 2015; **5**(8): e008424.

CHAPTER 6

Central line and peripheral line-associated bloodstream infection

Contents

Introduction

Intravascular devices are commonly used in hospital patients for medical treatment.[1] Point prevalence studies from the European Centre for Disease Prevention and Control (ECDC) reported central vascular device prevalence of 8% and peripheral vascular device prevalence of 47%.[2] A Japanese multicentred study identified central vascular device prevalence of 16% and peripheral vascular device prevalence of 30%,[3] while

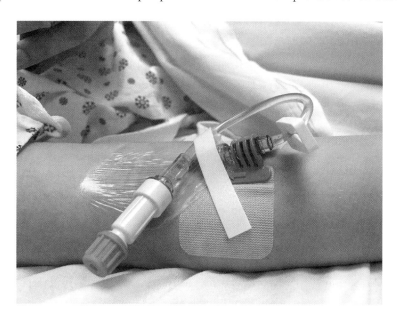

a multi-state study from the United States found a central vascular device prevalence of 18%.[4] A recent Australian point prevalent study found that 15% of adults in acute wards had a central vascular device, and 55% had a peripheral vascular device.[5]

Intravascular devices increase the risk of acquiring a bloodstream infection.[6] Device-related bloodstream infections cause increased morbidity and mortality and come at significant cost.[7,8] Although central venous catheters are less commonly used than peripheral catheters, it is estimated up to 15% of patients with a central venous catheter will experience a catheter-related complication.[9]

Internationally, extensive efforts have been directed towards reducing central line-associated bloodstream infections. These are commonly through the implementation of evidence-based strategies in the form of bundles.[10–12] Similar bundles exist for the prevention of peripheral line-associated bloodstream infections, but there is broad variation and uncertainty regarding effectiveness.[13]

The method of reporting bloodstream infection data related to vascular devices varies according to study methodology. Point prevalence study data from the ECDC report that 33% of bloodstream infections identified were central vascular device related, while 6% were peripheral vascular device related.[2] A similar multicentred study in Singapore identified that 21% of bloodstream infections were vascular device related.[14] In a large multicentred Spanish study, incidence of central vascular device bloodstream infections ranged from 0.01–0.14/1000 patient days and the peripheral vascular device bloodstream infections incidence was 0.05/1000 patient days.[15] In a large systematic review, the peripheral vascular device bloodstream infections pooled mean incidence of 0.5 per 1000 device days was reported.[6]

Definitions and context

The definitions of a central line and peripheral line bloodstream infection commonly first require the identification of a bloodstream infection with a positive microbiological blood culture, then applying clinical criteria. Following this, the application of further criteria can be used to determine association with a device. Examples of central catheter and peripheral catheter bloodstream infection definitions are provided in Table 6.1. For further and more detailed explanations and their applications, please refer to the source document referenced.

This chapter presents a collation and analysis of the three types of Australian healthcare-associated central line and peripheral line bloodstream infection data: 1. proportions of central line and peripheral line bloodstream infection hospital-acquired complication (HAC) for the period 1 July 2017 to 30 June 2019; 2. publicly available state and territory jurisdiction surveillance data for the period 1 July 2017 to 31 December 2018; and 3. peer-reviewed literature data for the period 1 January 2010 to 31 August 2019. Each of these potential data sources were interrogated to gain

Table 6.1 Examples of central line and peripheral line-associated bloodstream infections definitions

Country/ organisation	Subcategory	Overview of definition
Australia		No nationally agreed or defined surveillance definition
United States CDC NHSN[16]	Three pages of LCBI criteria	Primary bloodstream infection (BSI): A laboratory confirmed bloodstream infection (LCBI) that is not secondary to an infection at another body site
Europe (ECDC)[17]		<ul><li>Patient has at least one positive blood culture for a recognised pathogen OR</li><li>patient has at least one of the following signs or symptoms: fever (> 38°C), chills or hypotension and two positive blood cultures for a common skin contaminant (from two separate blood samples, usually within 48 hours).</li></ul>Skin contaminants = coagulase-negative staphylococci, *Micrococcus* spp., *Propionibacterium acnes*, *Bacillus* spp., *Corynebacterium* spp. Device-associated healthcare-associated infection (HAI) is a HAI in a patient with a (relevant) device that was used within the 48-hour period before onset of infection (even intermittently). The term 'device-associated' is only used for pneumonia, bloodstream infection and urinary tract infection (UTI). The 'relevant devices' are intubation, vascular (central/peripheral) catheter and urinary catheter, respectively. If the interval is longer than 48 hours, there must be compelling evidence that the infection was associated with device use. For catheter-associated UTI, the indwelling urinary catheter must have been in place within 7 days before positive laboratory results or signs and symptoms meeting criteria for UTI were evident. A bloodstream infection (BSI and secondary BSI) is always registered as a separate HAI with specification of the source in a separate field (peripheral or central catheter, other infection site—S-PUL, S-UTI, S-DIG, S-SSI, SSST, S-OTH); the only exceptions are a CRI3 (catheter-related bloodstream infection with microbiological documentation of the relationship between the vascular catheter and the BSI) and neonatal bloodstream infections: CRI3 and neonatal BSIs should not be reported twice in the point prevalence survey. Microbiologically confirmed catheter-related BSI should be reported as a CRI3. Neonatal bloodstream infections should be reported as NEO-LCBI or NEO-CNSB, together with BSI origin.

insight into the incidence of healthcare-associated central line and peripheral line bloodstream infection in Australia and the findings are presented below.

Findings

1. Healthcare-associated infection due to hospital-acquired complication (HAI HAC) data

Data on HAI HACs in Australia are collected by the Independent Hospital Pricing Authority (IHPA) but are not currently reported or publicly available. These data were provided upon request. The jurisdictions did not grant permission to publish the raw data but gave permission to report data by proportions. The number of HAI HACs central line and peripheral line-associated bloodstream infections are thus presented as a proportion. The raw data from which these proportions were calculated were provided by the IHPA.[18]

The burden of central line and peripheral line-associated bloodstream infections in Australian public hospitals, as identified by HAI HAC data, by state and territory, for 2017–2018 and 2018–2019 is presented in Table 6.2 and Figure 6.1. Over both time periods, 80% of reported central line and peripheral line-associated bloodstream infections occurred in New South Wales, Victoria and Queensland (the most populous states). Proportions of central line and peripheral line-associated bloodstream infections for each jurisdiction across the time periods were generally consistent.

Table 6.2 Nationwide distribution of HAC HAI central line and peripheral line-associated bloodstream infections by jurisdiction (%)

Jurisdiction	Timeframe	
	1 July 2017 – 30 June 2018	*1 July 2018 – 30 June 2019*
NSW	41.0	38.4
Vic.	17.8	18.6
Qld	21.0	22.7
SA	4.5	5.0
WA	10.7	9.6
Tas.	2.0	3.0
NT	1.1	0.7
ACT	1.8	2.1

Note: ACT = Australian Capital Territory. NSW = New South Wales. NT = Northern Territory. Qld = Queensland. SA = South Australia. Tas. = Tasmania. Vic. = Victoria. WA = Western Australia.
(Source: Compiled from IHPA data.)

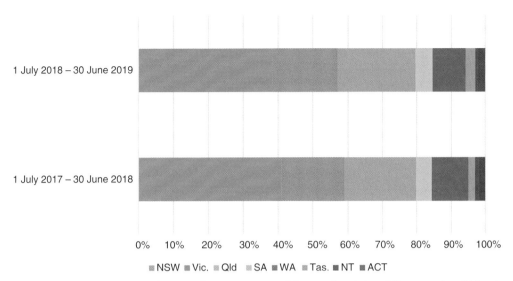

Figure 6.1 *Nationwide distribution of HAC HAI central line and peripheral line-associated bloodstream infections by jurisdiction (%)*

Note: ACT = Australian Capital Territory. NSW = New South Wales. NT = Northern Territory. Qld = Queensland. SA = South Australia. Tas. = Tasmania. Vic. = Victoria. WA = Western Australia.

(Source: Compiled from IHPA data.)

2. Jurisdictional HAI data

Central and peripheral line infection data by jurisdiction is presented in Table 6.3. Not all jurisdictions had data available.

3. Peer-reviewed literature data

Table 6.4 summarises the findings from articles identified from the peer-reviewed literature. Three of the four studies identified were conducted in Victoria. All studies used HSN CDC definitions for CLABSI.

The definition of the HAI applied in each of the studies identified in the literature is listed in Table 6.5.

Synthesis and summary

National data on device-associated bloodstream infections in Australia is lacking. Despite the associated significant morbidity and mortality, unlike other developed countries, there is no nationally coordinated effort to define or describe this condition in Australia.

Table 6.3 Central and peripheral line infection data by jurisdiction

Year	ACT	NSW	NT	Qld	SA[19]	Tas.[20]	Vic.[21]	WA[22]
2017–2018	–	–	–	–	2017: Intravascular line associated BSI n = 135. Of these, n = 98 were central line associated.	44% of HA-SAB were related to IV devices.	ICU (excludes neonatal) CLABSI: Major teaching hospitals 0.83/1000 line days Other hospitals 0.48/1000 line days.	Haemodialysis associated BSI: • cuffed catheter 0.98 (95% CI: 0.69–1.38) • non-cuffed catheter 0.00 (95% CI: 0.00–6.23) Adult ICU CLABSI: 0.33/1000 line days. Haematology CLABSI: 0.59/1000 line days. Oncology CLABSI: 0.07/1000 line days.
2018–2019	–	–	–	–	2018: Intravascular line-associated BSI n = 198. Of these 149 were central line associated.	–	–	–

Note: – indicates data was not available. ACT = Australian Capital Territory. NSW = New South Wales. NT = Northern Territory. Qld = Queensland. SA = South Australia. Tas. = Tasmania. Vic. = Victoria. WA = Western Australia.

Table 6.4 Data on central and peripheral line infections identified from literature research

Lead author	Year	Location (no. of hospitals)	Year(s) study was undertaken	Population	Type of HAI monitored	Key finding
Campbell[23]	2019	WA (1)	2014–2015	11,774 processed blood culture bottles from PICU	CLABSIs	73/122 cases of HA-BSI were HA-CLABSI
Spelman[24]	2017	Vic. (26)	2010–2013	ICU-admitted patients	CLABSIs	Aggregate annual CLABSI rates. 2010: 1.72/1000 CVC days (95% CI: 1.40–2.08) 2011: 1.37/1000 CVC days (95% CI: 1.08–1.70) 2012: 1.00/1000 CVC days (95% CI: 0.75–1.30) 2013: 0.93/1000 CVC days (95% CI: 0.69–1.24)
Wong[25]	2016	Vic. (1)	2008–2014	ICU	Central line-associated BSI	1.12/1000 ICU CVC-days; 36 per 1000 ICU CVC days
Worth[26]	2019	Vic. (4 neonates, 1 paeds)	2009–2016	ICU paeds and neonates	CLABSI PLABSI	CLABSI neonates 2.2/1000 (95% CI: 1.9–2.5) CLABSI paeds 2.2/1000 (95% CI: 1.8–2.7) PLABSI neonates 0.67/1000 (95% CI: 0.54–0.82) PLABSI paeds not recorded

Note: BSI = bloodstream infection. CLABSI = central line-associated bloodstream infection. CVC = central venous catheter. HA = healthcare-associated. ICU = intensive care unit. PICU = paediatric intensive care unit. Vic. = Victoria. WA = Western Australia.

Table 6.5 HAI definitions used in the identified studies

Lead author	Year	HAI definition used
Campbell[23]	2019	Health Infection Surveillance Western Australia definitions that concur with NHSN CDC definitions were used for CLABSI
Spelman[24]	2017	CDC NHSN criteria for CLABSI: when patient had recognised pathogen in one or more cultures and the organism wasn't related to infection at another site, or patient had one or more of fever, chills, hypotension, a common commensal organism in two or more blood cultures from separate occasions and positive results not related to infection at another site
Wong[25]	2016	CLABSI was defined according to the CDC NHSN surveillance criteria; an ICU-acquired CLABSI was defined as any CLABSI occurring in ICU or within 48 hours of discharge
Worth[26]	2019	CDC NHSN criteria for CLABSI

Note: CDC = Centers for Disease Control and Prevention. CLABSI = central line-associated bloodstream infection. HAI = healthcare-associated infection. NHSN = National Healthcare Safety Network. ICU = intensive care unit.

HAC data are administrative data collected by hospitals originally designed for accounting purposes. Multiple studies have demonstrated their unreliability in identifying HAIs.[27] As well as unreliability, the HAC data provided here are unable to be interpreted given the lack of both numerator and denominator data. The data provided indicates that more HAC-related device-associated bloodstream infections data are reported from the more populous states, which is to be expected given there are more hospitals in the larger states.

Four states publicly report device-related bloodstream infection data. There is no specific data relating to peripheral vascular device bloodstream infections, and only Western Australia and Victoria report similar data on adult intensive care unit central line bloodstream infections. The Victorian data include some private hospitals as well as public hospitals. Rates of central and peripheral line bloodstream infections are also provided for neonatal intensive care units but are complicated because they are broken down by birth weight, as per CDC methodology. Tasmanian data are only provided in relation to HCA-SAB related to IV devices with no indication of the type or proportion of each IV device associated with the infection.

Data from the peer-reviewed literature are more informative and homogeneous, though restricted to research from Western Australia and Victoria. Although all four studies used definitions derived from the CDC, the West Australian study population was a paediatric ICU population, two Victorian study populations were adult ICU, and another paediatric and neonatal ICU, which may explain some differences in rates.

Despite well-validated international definitions and surveillance methodology for CLABSI, the common use of such data for performance measurement and a fundamental surveillance activity characteristic of mature infection prevention programs, there is very little data available in Australia. Some states appear to have well-established processes in place for surveillance and reporting; however, there is little uniformity nationally.

References

1. Alexandrou E, Ray-Barruel G, Carr PJ, et al. Use of Short Peripheral Intravenous Catheters: Characteristics, Management, and Outcomes Worldwide. *J Hosp Med* 2018; **13**(5).
2. European Centre for Disease Prevention and Control. Point prevalence survey of healthcare-associated infections and antimicrobial use in European acute care hospitals. Stockholm: ECDC, 2013.
3. Morioka H, Hirabayashi A, Iguchi M, et al. The first point prevalence survey of healthcare–associated infection and antimicrobial use in a Japanese university hospital: A pilot study. *Am J Infect Control* 2016; **44**(7): e119–23.
4. Magill SS, Edwards JR, Bamberg W, et al. Multistate point-prevalence survey of health care-associated infections. *N Engl J Med* 2014; **370**(13): 1198–208.
5. Russo PL, Stewardson A, Cheng AC, et al. The prevalence of healthcare-associated infections among adult inpatients at nineteen large Australian acute-care public hospitals: a point prevalence survey. *Antimicrob Resist Infect Control* 2019; **8**(114).
6. Maki DG, Kluger DM, Crnic CJ. The risk of bloodstream infection in adults with different intravascular devices: a systematic review of 200 published prospective studies. *Mayo Clin Proc* 2006; **81**: 1159–71.
7. Goudie A, Dynan L, Brady PW, et al. Attributable cost and length of stay for central line-associated bloodstream infections. *Pediatrics* 2014; **133**(6): e1525–32.
8. Kaye KS, Marchaim D, Chen TY, et al. Effect of nosocomial bloodstream infections on mortality, length of stay, and hospital costs in older adults. *J Am Geriatr Soc* 2014; **62**(2): 306–11.
9. Smith RN, Nolan JP. Central venous catheters. *BMJ* 2013; **347**: f6570.
10. Furuya EY, Dick AW, Herzig CT, et al. Central Line-Associated Bloodstream Infection Reduction and Bundle Compliance in Intensive Care Units: A National Study. *Infect Control Hosp Epidemiol* 2016; **37**(7): 805–10.
11. Lai CC, Cia CT, Chiang HT, et al. Implementation of a national bundle care program to reduce central line-associated bloodstream infections in intensive care units in Taiwan. *J Microbiol Immunol Infect* 2018; **51**(5): 666–71.
12. Render ML, Hasselbeck R, Freyberg RW, et al. Reduction of central line infections in Veterans Administration intensive care units: an observational cohort using a central infrastructure to support learning and improvement. *BMJ Qual Saf* 2011; **20**(8): 725–32.
13. Ray-Barruel G, Xu H, Marsh N, et al. Effectiveness of insertion and maintenance bundles in preventing peripheral intravenous catheter-related complications and bloodstream infection in hospital patients: A systematic review. *Infect Dis Health* 2019; **24**(3): 152–68.
14. Cai Y, Venkatachalam I, Tee NW, et al. Prevalence of Healthcare-Associated Infections and Antimicrobial Use Among Adult Inpatients in Singapore Acute-Care Hospitals: Results From the First National Point Prevalence Survey. *Clin Infect Dis* 2017; **64**(suppl_2): S61–7.
15. Freixas N, Bella F, Limón E, et al. Impact of a multimodal intervention to reduce bloodstream infections related to vascular catheters in non-ICU wards: a multicentre study. *Clin Microbiol Infect* 2013; **19**(9): 838–44.
16. Centers for Disease Control and Prevention. Bloodstream Infection Event (Central Line-Associated Bloodstream Infection and Non-central Line Associated Bloodstream Infection). 2020.
17. European Centre for Disease Prevention and Control. Point prevalence survey of healthcare-associated infections and antimicrobial use in European acute care hospitals—protocol version 5.3. Stockholm: ECDC, 2016.

18. Independent Hospital Pricing Authority. Healthcare-associated infections Hospital-acquired complication (HAI HAC) data. In: Independent Hospital Pricing Authority, editor. Sydney, Australia: Independent Hospital Pricing Authority; 2020.

19. Cope C. South Australian Healthcare-associated Infection Surveillance Program: Bloodstream Infection Annual Report 2018. In: Infection Control Service CDCB, editor. Adelaide, South Australia: SA Department for Health and Wellbeing; 2019. p. 25.

20. Wilson F, Anderson T, Wells A. Tasmanian Acute Public Hospitals Healthcare Associated Infection Report No 38 – Annual Report 2017–18. In: Services DoHaH, editor. Hobart: Department of Health and Human Services, Tasmania; 2018. p. 43.

21. Department of Health and Human Services, The University of Melbourne, The Royal Melbourne Hospital, The Peter Doherty Institute for Infection and Immunity. Healthcare-associated infection in Victoria: Surveillance report for 2016–17 and 2017–18. Melbourne, Australia, 2018.

22. Communicable Disease Control Directorate. Healthcare Infection Surveillance Western Australia: Annual Report 2017–18. Perth, Western Australia, 2018.

23. Campbell AJ, Blyth CC, Hewison CJ, et al. Lessons learned from a hospital-wide review of blood stream infections for paediatric central line-associated blood stream infection prevention. *J Paediatr Child Health* 2019; **55**(6): 690–4.

24. Spelman T, Pilcher DV, Cheng AC, et al. Central line-associated bloodstream infections in Australian ICUs: evaluating modifiable and non-modifiable risks in Victorian healthcare facilities. *Epidemiol Infect* 2017; **145**(14): 3047–55.

25. Wong SW, Gantner D, McGloughlin S, et al. The influence of intensive care unit-acquired central line-associated bloodstream infection on in-hospital mortality: A single-center risk-adjusted analysis. *Am J Infect Control* 2016; **44**(5): 587–92.

26. Worth LJ, Daley AJ, Spelman T, et al. Central and peripheral line-associated bloodstream infections in Australian neonatal and paediatric intensive care units: findings from a comprehensive Victorian surveillance network, 2008–2016. *J Hosp Infect* 2018; **99**(1): 55–61.

27. van Mourik MSM, van Duijn PJ, Moons KGM, et al. Accuracy of administrative data for surveillance of healthcare-associated infections: a systematic review. *BMJ Open* 2015; **5**(8).

CHAPTER 7

Multi-resistant organisms

Contents

Introduction

There are various multi–resistant organisms (MROs) that cause morbidity and mortality in healthcare facilities. MROs can lead to increased hospital stay and/or admission to intensive care units. Driven by the increased and often inappropriate use of antimicrobials, the growing incidence of MROs is a worldwide problem. Of particular importance

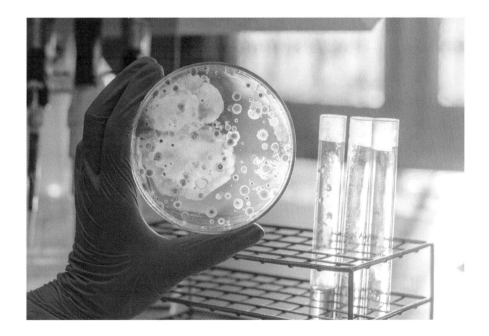

are methicillin-resistant *Staphylococcus aureus* (MRSA),[1,2] vancomycin-resistant Enterococci (VRE),[3] multi-resistant Gram-negative bacilli (MRGN),[4] including the carbapenemase-producing *Enterobacterales*,[5] and the fungal pathogen, *Candida auris*.[6] The United States Centers for Disease Control and Prevention (CDC) estimates that 2.8 million antimicrobial-resistant (AMR) infections occur in the United States every year, resulting in more than 35,000 deaths.[7] The economic burden of MROs is staggering and can cost approximately US$2–3 billion every year.[8–12] One case of MRSA was reported to cost healthcare facilities up to US$31,338 for treatment and management of the infection.[13]

Definitions and context

Antimicrobial susceptibility of an organism is determined by their susceptibility or resistance to an antimicrobial agent. These susceptibility categories are determined through clinical breakpoints (i.e. the set concentration of an antimicrobial which defines whether a microorganism is susceptible or resistant to the antimicrobial). These are updated yearly by the European Committee on Antimicrobial and Susceptibility Testing (EUCAST)[14,15] and the Clinical and Laboratory Standards Institute (CLSI). Clinical breakpoints set by CLSI are not publicly available.

National strategies to target AMR in Australia have been outlined in *Australia's National Antimicrobial Resistance Strategy–2020 and Beyond*.[16] In a bid to combat AMR, the Australian Government has taken the 'One Health' approach by recognising the linkages between humans, animals, plants and the environment, and has called for interdisciplinary collaborations across private and public sectors, at local, national and global levels, to tackle AMR. In Australia, the Antimicrobial Use and Resistance in Australia (AURA) Surveillance System was established by the Australian Commission on Safety and Quality in Health Care (ACSQHC) to provide a nationally coordinated system for surveillance of antimicrobial resistance (AMR) and use of antimicrobials.[17]

Findings

This report presents a collation and analysis of the three types of Australian data for multi-resistant organism infections: 1. proportions of hospital-acquired complication (HAC) data for the period 1 July 2017 to 30 June 2019; 2. publicly available state and territory jurisdiction surveillance data for the period between 1 July 2017 and 31 August 2019; and 3. peer-reviewed literature data for the period 1 January 2010 to 31 August 2019. Each of these potential data sources was interrogated to gain insight into the incidence of multi-resistant organism infections in Australia and the findings are presented on the following pages.

1. Healthcare-associated infection due to hospital-acquired complication (HAI HAC) data

Data on healthcare-associated infection (HAI) HACs in Australia are collected by the Independent Hospital Pricing Authority (IHPA) but are not currently reported or publicly available. These data were provided upon request. The jurisdictions did not grant permission to publish the raw data but gave permission to report data by proportions. The number of HAI HACs MROs are thus presented as a proportion. The raw data from which these proportions were calculated were provided by the IHPA.[18]

The burden of MROs in Australian public hospitals, as identified by HAI HAC data, by state and territory for 2017–2018 and 2018–2019, is presented in Table 7.1 and Fig. 7.1. Over both time periods, 82% of reported MROs occurred in New South Wales, Victoria and Queensland (the most populous states). Proportions of MROs (%) in the jurisdictions over the time periods were generally consistent.

2. Jurisdictional HAI data

MRO data by jurisdiction is presented in Table 7.2. Not all jurisdictions had data available.

3. Peer-reviewed literature data

There was no specific peer-reviewed literature identified as part of the literature review search. The identification of specific multi-resistant infection was outside the scope of the search strategy employed. Where multi-resistant infections were identified

Table 7.1 Nationwide distribution of HAC HAI MROs by jurisdiction (%)

Jurisdiction	Timeline	
	1 July 2017 – 30 June 2018	*1 July 2018 – 30 June 2019*
NSW	29.2	28.3
Vic.	30.6	33.6
Qld	21.7	20.3
SA	5.3	4.2
WA	7.9	7.6
Tas.	2.2	2.6
NT	1.4	1.4
ACT	1.6	1.9

Note: ACT = Australian Capital Territory. NSW = New South Wales. NT = Northern Territory. Qld = Queensland.
   SA = South Australia. Tas. = Tasmania. Vic. = Victoria. WA = Western Australia.
(Source: Compiled from IHPA data.)

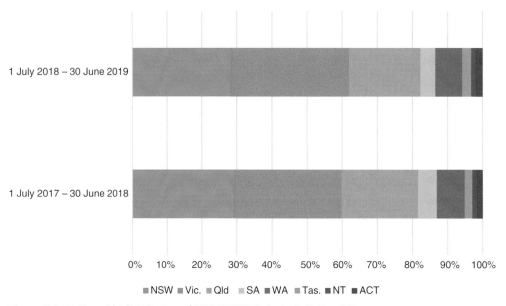

Figure 7.1 *Nationwide distribution of HAC HAI MROs by jurisdiction (%)*
Note: ACT = Australian Capital Territory. NSW = New South Wales. NT = Northern Territory. Qld = Queensland.
SA = South Australia. Tas. = Tasmania. Vic. = Victoria. WA = Western Australia.
(Source: Compiled from IHPA data.)

as part of other infections (e.g. bloodstream infections), these are contained within the respective chapters of this text.

4. Additional considerations

The ACSQHC administers the AURA Surveillance System, a voluntary system with no requirement for state or territory organisations to participate or provide data.[28] The reported strategy for the AURA Surveillance System is to increase participation in each of the surveillance components to maximise geographic coverage, as well as coverage of the community and acute sectors, and both the private and public sectors.[28] The approach is also intended to enable the collection methods, analyses and understanding of any limitations when using the data to be refined over time. AURA provides data and analyses on patterns and trends in resistance for priority organisms to key antimicrobials in acute care, aged care homes and the community.[28] Resistance data are collected for priority organisms across four sets of organisms. AURA 2019 provides resistance data for the priority organisms:

- *Acinetobacter baumannii*
- *Enterobacterales*

Table 7.2 Publicly available jurisdictional hospital-identified multi-resistant organism data for 2017/2018/2019

MRO	ACT	NSW	NT	Qld	SA[19,20]	Tas.[21]	Vic.[22]	WA[23-27]
Carbapenemase-producing *Enterobacteriaceae* (CPE)	—	—	—	—	—		2018 162 cases 2019 to September 204 cases	2017–2018 44 isolates 2018–2019 Q3 6 cases 2018–2019 Q4 6 cases 2019–2020 Q1 11 cases 2019/20 Q2 17 cases
MRSA HAI	—	—	—	—	**2017–2018 MRSA HA-BSI** 0.16/10,000 bed days **2018 MRSA infections** ICU sterile site 0.0 per 10,000 bed days ICU non-sterile site 0.59 per 10,000 bed days Non-ICU sterile site 0.22 per 10,000 bed days Non-ICU non-sterile site 0.67 per 10,000 bed days Total inpatient 0.89 per 10,000 bed days	MRSA bacteraemia numbers only 2017 6 cases 2018 3 cases	2017–2018 MRSA: HA-SAB (MRSA) =0.11/10,000 OBD	**MRSA HAI 2017–2018** ICU sterile site 0.12 per 10,000 bed days ICU non-sterile site 1.58 per 10,000 bed days Non-ICU sterile site 0.25 per 10,000 bed days Non-ICU non-sterile site 0.78 per 10,000 bed days Total inpatient 1.06 per 10,000 bed days 2018–2019 Q2 Total inpatient 0.92/10,000 bed days

Continued

Table 7.2 Publicly available jurisdictional hospital-identified multi-resistant organism data for 2017/2018/2019—cont'd

MRO	ACT	NSW	NT	Qld	SA[19,20]	Tas.[21]	Vic.[22]	WA[23-27]
Vancomycin-resistant Enterococci (VRE)	—	—	—	—	Infections 2017 0.69 per 10,000 bed days 2018 0.28 per 10,000 bed days	VRE infections numbers only 2017 13 cases 2018 31 cases	—	2018–2019 Q4 Total inpatient 0.76/10,000 bed days 2019–2020 Q1 Total inpatient 0.66 per 10,000 bed days 2019–2020 Q2 Total inpatient 0.75 per 10,000 bed days 2017–2018 Sterile site 0.1 per 10,000 bed days 2018–2019 Q3 Sterile site 1 case HAI 2018–2019 Q4 Sterile site 1 case HAI 2019–2020 Q1 Sterile site 1 case HAI 2019–2020 Q2 Sterile site 1 case HAI

MRGNs				Healthcare-associated critical antimicrobial resistance acquisitions	
–	–	–	–		–
–					–

MRGNS multidrug-resistant *Pseudomonas aeruginosa* (MRPAER), extended beta-lactamase producers (ESBL), carbapenem- resistant *Acinetobacter* species and Enterobacterales (CRGNB), plasmid-mediated Amp C beta-lactamase producers (AMPC) and metallo-beta-lactamase producers (MBL).

Total acquisitions
2017
3
2018
4

Note: Vic. CPE: infection or colonisation. A case is defined by the organism (not patient) and the resistance genes. – indicates that data was not available. ACT = Australian Capital Territory. NSW = New South Wales. NT = Northern Territory. OBD = occupied bed days. Qld = Queensland. SA = South Australia. Tas. = Tasmania. Vic. = Victoria. WA = Western Australia.

- *Enterococcus* species
- *Mycobacterium tuberculosis*
- *Neisseria gonorrhoeae*
- *Neisseria meningitidis*
- *Pseudomonas aeruginosa*
- *Salmonella* species
- *Shigella* species
- *Staphylococcus aureus*
- *Streptococcus agalactiae*
- *Streptococcus pneumoniae*
- *Streptococcus pyogenes*.

The AURA Surveillance System draws on both passive and targeted surveillance data from a range of existing agencies, namely the Australian Group on Antimicrobial Resistance (AGAR), the National Alert System for Critical Antimicrobial Resistances (CARAlert), the Australian Passive AMR Surveillance (APAS), the National Neisseria Network (NNN), the National Notifiable Diseases Surveillance System (NNDSS) and Sullivan Nicolaides Pathology (SNP).[28] These agencies provide data to the AURA Surveillance System as outlined in Table 7.3.[28]

Data collected and reported in AURA are laboratory-based and do not denote in and of themselves a HAI. Denominator data for MROs are not available for all the AURA partner programs for a range of reported reasons, all based on the intended purpose of the data and subsequent analyses. Estimates of the burden of resistance, overall and by syndrome, are prepared to determine the extent of the problem whereas estimates of the proportion of resistant isolates for each species are used to determine the probability of primary treatment failure and to inform guidelines about primary therapeutic choices.[28]

Synthesis and summary

Despite the criticality of antimicrobial resistance to safety and quality in healthcare, there is very little publicly available data reporting rates of multi-drug resistant infection. HAC data are administrative data collected by hospitals, originally designed for accounting purposes. Multiple studies have demonstrated their unreliability in identifying HAI.[29] As well as unreliability, the HAC data provided here are unable to be interpreted given the lack of both numerator and denominator data.

Publicly reported jurisdictional data on MROs is sparse with no data available for Queensland, New South Wales, the Australian Capital Territory and the Northern Territory. Where jurisdictional data are publicly available, organisms and surveillance periods vary. Carbapenemase-producing *Enterobacterales* (CPE) data are reported as cases by year by Victoria, cases by quarter by Tasmania and isolates by year by Western

Table 7.3 Data sources for multi-resistant organism within the AURA Surveillance System[28]

Subject and type of surveillance	Data source	Type of data	Setting	Coverage
• Antimicrobial resistance • Targeted • Community	Australian Group on Antimicrobial Resistance	Rates of resistance, 30-day all-cause mortality	Australian public and private hospitals (community onset)	• All states and territories • 2016: 28 laboratories servicing 32 hospitals and their communities • 2017: 29 laboratories servicing 36 hospitals and their communities
	CARAlert	Rates of resistance for priority organisms	Australian general practices, aged care homes, community health services and hospital non-admitted care services	• National • 28 confirming laboratories
	National Notifiable Diseases Surveillance System	Rates of resistance and trends for *Mycobacterium tuberculosis*	Australian general practices, community health services and hospital non-admitted care services	• National • 5 reference laboratories
	National Neisseria Network	Rates of resistance and trends for *Neisseria gonorrhoeae* and *Neisseria meningitidis*	Australian general practices, community health services and hospital non-admitted care services	• National • 9 reference laboratories
• Antimicrobial resistance • Targeted • Hospital	Australian Group on Antimicrobial Resistance	Rates of resistance, 30-day all-cause mortality	Australian public and private hospitals (hospital onset)	National 2016: 28 laboratories servicing 32 hospitals 2017: 29 laboratories servicing 36 hospitals
	CARAlert	Rates of resistance for priority organisms	Australian public and private hospitals	National 28 confirming laboratories

Continued

Table 7.3 Data sources for multi-resistant organism within the AURA Surveillance System—cont'd

Subject and type of surveillance	Data source	Type of data	Setting	Coverage
• Antimicrobial resistance • Passive • Community	Australian Passive AMR Surveillance	Rates of resistance	Community and aged care homes	Each of the laboratory services provides access to a range of resistance testing for primary care and non-admitted hospital patients; laboratories estimated that testing for the community sector represents 30–85% of their workload
	Sullivan Nicolaides Pathology	Rates of resistance	Community and aged care homes	Queensland and northern New South Wales
• Antimicrobial resistance • Passive • Hospital	Australian Passive AMR Surveillance	Rates of resistance	Australian Capital Territory, New South Wales, Queensland, South Australia, Tasmania, Victoria, Western Australia	All Queensland public hospitals; Mater Pathology Brisbane (selected private hospitals, Queensland); all public hospitals and private hospitals in South Australia; selected public hospitals and health services in the Australian Capital Territory, New South Wales, Tasmania, Victoria and Western Australia
	Sullivan Nicolaides Pathology	Rates of resistance	Queensland and northern New South Wales	Queensland and northern New South Wales

(Source: 2019 AURA Report,[28] p. 17)

Australia. Healthcare-associated MRSA infections are reported by site by South Australia and Western Australia; however, South Australia reports by calendar year for 2018 and Western Australia reports by financial year for 2017–2018.

Although VRE data are reported by South Australia, Tasmania, Victoria and Western Australia, once again there are variations in how these data are reported, preventing comparison. Based on the data that are available, the rate of VRE infections in South Australia decreased between 2017 and 2018, while the number of cases in Tasmania increased from 13 in 2017 to 31 in 2018. In Western Australia the number of sterile site cases remained static in the periods reported.

The only jurisdictional data available on MRGN organisms was published by South Australia, identifying 3 cases in 2017 and 4 cases in 2018. Due to the variability in reporting, it is not possible to compare interjurisdictional rates of MRO infection.

Data collected and reported via AURA are predominantly laboratory-based and are not specifically defined as HAIs (noting some subsets of the AURA report may contain HAI data). The purpose of AURA is to report resistance, not specifically report on HAI incidence or prevalence.

References

1. Dulon M, Haamann F, Peters C, et al. MRSA prevalence in European healthcare settings: a review. *BMC Infect Dis* 2011; **11**: 138.
2. Worth LJ, Spelman T, Bull AL, et al. *Staphylococcus aureus* bloodstream infection in Australian hospitals: findings from a Victorian surveillance system. *Med J Aust* 2014; **200**(5): 282–4.
3. Mutters NT, Mersch-Sundermann V, Mutters R, et al. Control of the spread of vancomycin-resistant Enterococci in hospitals: epidemiology and clinical relevance. *Dtsch Arztebl Int* 2013; **110**(43): 725–31.
4. Chia PY, Sengupta S, Kukreja A, et al. The role of hospital environment in transmissions of multidrug-resistant gram-negative organisms. *Antimicrob Resist Infect Control* 2020; **9**(1): 29.
5. Brett JA, Johnson SA, Cameron DRM, et al. Carbapenemase-producing Enterobacteriaceae in Australian hospitals: outcome of point-prevalence screening in high-risk wards. *J Hosp Infect* 2019; **101**(2): 163–6.
6. Chowdhary A, Voss A, Meis JF. Multidrug-resistant *Candida auris*: 'new kid on the block' in hospital-associated infections? *J Hosp Infect* 2016; **94**(3): 209–12.
7. Centers for Disease Control and Prevention. Antibiotic resistance threats in the United States, 2019. 2019.
8. Dadgostar P. Antimicrobial Resistance: Implications and Costs. *Infect Drug Resist* 2019; **12**: 3903–10.
9. Shrestha P, Cooper BS, Coast J, et al. Enumerating the economic cost of antimicrobial resistance per antibiotic consumed to inform the evaluation of interventions affecting their use. *Antimicrob Resist Infect Control* 2018; **7**: 98.
10. Naylor NR, Atun R, Zhu N, et al. Estimating the burden of antimicrobial resistance: a systematic literature review. *Antimicrob Resist Infect Control* 2018; **7**: 58.
11. Thorpe KE, Joski P, Johnston KJ. Antibiotic-Resistant Infection Treatment Costs Have Doubled Since 2002, Now Exceeding $2 Billion Annually. *Health Aff* 2018; **37**(4): 662–9.
12. Gandra S, Barter DM, Laxminarayan R. Economic burden of antibiotic resistance: how much do we really know? *Clin Microbiol Infect* 2014; **20**(10): 973–80.

13. Wozniak TM, Barnsbee L, Lee XJ, et al. Using the best available data to estimate the cost of antimicrobial resistance: a systematic review. *Antimicrob Resist Infect Control* 2019; **8**: 26.

14. European Committee on Antimicrobial Susceptibility Testing. The European Committee on Antimicrobial Susceptibility Testing. Breakpoint tables for interpretation of MICs and zone diameters, 2020.

15. European Committee on Antimicrobial Susceptibility Testing. The European Committee on Antimicrobial Susceptibility Testing. Breakpoint tables for interpretation of MICs for antifungal agents, version 10.0, 2020.

16. Australian Government. Australia's National Antimicrobial Resistance Strategy–2020 and Beyond In: Department of Health and Department of Water, Agriculture and the Environment, editors. Commonwealth of Australia; 2020. p. 18.

17. Australian Commission on Safety and Quality in Health Care. Antimicrobial Use and Resistance in Australia Surveillance System. 2020. https://www.safetyandquality.gov.au/our-work/antimicrobial-resistance/antimicrobial-use-and-resistance-australia-surveillance-system (accessed 28 May 2020).

18. Independent Hospital Pricing Authority. Healthcare-associated infections Hospital-acquired complication (HAI HAC) data. In: Independent Hospital Pricing Authority, editor. Sydney, Australia: Independent Hospital Pricing Authority; 2020.

19. Cope C. South Australian Healthcare-associated Infection Surveillance Program: Multidrug-resistant Organisms Annual Report 2018. In: Infection Control Service CDCB, editor. Adelaide, South Australia: SA Department for Health and Wellbeing; 2019. p. 19.

20. Cope C. South Australian Healthcare-associated Infection Surveillance Program: Bloodstream Infection Annual Report 2018. In: Infection Control Service CDCB, editor. Adelaide, South Australia: SA Department for Health and Wellbeing; 2019. p. 25.

21. Department of Health, Tasmanian Government. Healthcare associated infection surveillance. January 2018; 2020. https://www.dhhs.tas.gov.au/publichealth/tasmanian_infection_prevention_and_control_unit/HAI_Surveillance (accessed 12 June 2020).

22. Department of Health and Human Services, The University of Melbourne, The Royal Melbourne Hospital, The Peter Doherty Institute for Infection and Immunity. Healthcare-associated infection in Victoria: Surveillance report for 2016–17 and 2017–18. Melbourne, Australia, 2018.

23. Communicable Disease Control Directorate. Healthcare Infection Surveillance Western Australia (HISWA) Quarterly Report: Quarter 1 2019–20 Data for July to September 2019; 2019.

24. Communicable Disease Control Directorate. Healthcare Infection Surveillance Western Australia (HISWA) Quarterly Report: Quarter 2 2019–20 Data for October to December 2019; 2020.

25. Communicable Disease Control Directorate. Healthcare Infection Surveillance Western Australia (HISWA) Quarterly Report: Quarter 3 2018–19 Data for January to March 2019; 2019.

26. Communicable Disease Control Directorate. Healthcare Infection Surveillance Western Australia (HISWA) Quarterly Report: Quarter 4 2018–19 Data for April to June 2019; 2019.

27. Communicable Disease Control Directorate. Healthcare Infection Surveillance Western Australia: Annual Report 2017–18. Perth, Western Australia, 2018.

28. Australian Commission on Safety and Quality in Health Care. AURA 2019: third Australian report on antimicrobial use and resistance in human health. Sydney: Australian Commission on Safety and Quality in Health Care; 2019.

29. van Mourik MSM, van Duijn PJ, Moons KGM, et al. Accuracy of administrative data for surveillance of healthcare-associated infections: a systematic review. *BMJ Open* 2015; **5**(8).

CHAPTER 8

Infection associated with prosthetics and implantable devices

Contents

Introduction

Implantable devices such as those used in cardiac surgery are designed to save the life of a patient while prostheses such as those used in joint replacement surgery are designed to improve the quality of life for the patient.[1,2]

The implantable device or prosthesis is designed to remain in the body permanently and can include cardiac pacemakers, joint prostheses, breast implants, ventricular shunts

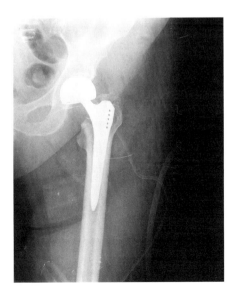

and non–human heart valves.[3] Infection associated with prosthetics and implantable devices is a major complication resulting in morbidity and mortality. Although the infection rates are reported to be low, the impact of infections is significant such as those associated with prosthetic joint replacements where adverse outcomes can range from impaired function to amputation and sepsis.[4,5] Associated with these unintended consequences for the patient are increased healthcare costs, increased length of hospital stay, additional surgery and potentially long–term antibiotic use. Furthermore, the number of procedures performed each year involving implantable devices and prostheses is substantial. For example, more than 600,000 knee and almost 300,000 hip replacement procedures are performed annually in the United States alone.[1–3,6]

Such is the impact of infection associated with implantable devices and prostheses, prevention strategies have extended beyond the usual raft of infection prevention and control initiatives, and a range of engineering controls have been trialled with variable success.[7,8] The effect of any strategy aimed at preventing infection can only be determined on the basis of robust data derived from surveillance initiatives. Implantation of these devices and prostheses requires a surgical procedure and therefore surveillance of infections associated with these devices is often a subset of surgical site surveillance.

This chapter presents the publicly available Australian data on infections associated with prosthetics and implantable devices.

Definitions and context

The definition of an infection associated with prosthetics and implantable devices varies according to country; however, examples of prosthetics and implantable devices surveillance definitions are provided in Table 8.1. For further and more detailed explanations and their applications, please refer to the source document referenced.

Findings

This chapter presents a collation and analysis of the three types of Australian data for infections associated with prosthetics and implantable devices: 1. proportions of hospital–acquired complication (HAC) data for the period 1 July 2017 to 30 June 2019; 2. publicly available state and territory jurisdiction surveillance data for the period 1 July 2017 to 30 June 2018; and 3. peer–reviewed literature data for the period 1 January 2010 to 31 August 2019. Each of these potential data sources was interrogated to gain insight into the incidence of healthcare–associated infections (HAIs) associated with prosthetics and implantable devices in Australia and the findings are presented on the following pages.

Table 8.1 Examples of implantable device and prostheses infection definitions

Country/ organisation	Subcategory	Overview of definition
Australia		No nationally agreed or defined surveillance definition.
United States CDC NHSN[3]★	Superficial incisional SSI (further definitions are provided in relation to primary incision site and secondary incision site)	Date of event occurs within 30 days after any NHSN operative procedure (where day 1 = the procedure date) AND involves on skin and subcutaneous tissue of the incision AND patient has at least **_one_** of the following: a. purulent drainage from the superficial incision. b. organism(s) identified from an aseptically obtained specimen from the superficial incision or subcutaneous tissue by a culture or non-culture-based microbiologic testing method which is performed for purposes of clinical diagnosis or treatment (e.g. not Active Surveillance Culture/Testing [ACT/AST]). c. superficial incision that is deliberately opened by a surgeon, physician★ or physician designee and culture or non-culture-based testing of the superficial incision or subcutaneous tissue is not performed AND patient has at least one of the following signs or symptoms: localised pain or tenderness; localised swelling; erythema; or heat. d. Diagnosis of a superficial incisional SSI by a physician★ or physician designee.

Continued

Table 8.1 Examples of implantable device and prostheses infection definitions—cont'd

Country/ organisation	Subcategory	Overview of definition
	Deep incisional SSI (further definitions are provided in relation to deep primary incision site and deep secondary incision site)	The date of the event occurs within 30 or 90 days after the NHSN operative procedure (where day 1 = the procedure date) according to the list in Table 2 [*of the source document*] (specific procedures are listed) AND involves deep soft tissues of the incision (e.g. fascia and muscle layers) AND patient has at least one of the following: a. purulent drainage from the deep incision b. a deep incision that spontaneously dehisces, or is deliberately opened or aspirated by a surgeon, physician★ or physician designee AND organism(s) identified from the deep soft tissues of the incision by a culture or non-culture-based microbiologic testing method which is performed for purposes of clinical diagnosis or treatment (e.g. not Active Surveillance Culture/Testing [ACT/ AST]) or culture or non-culture-based microbiologic testing method is not performed. A culture or non-culture-based test from the deep soft tissues of the incision that has a negative finding does not meet this criterion AND patient has at least **_one_** of the following signs or symptoms: fever (> 38°C); localised pain or tenderness c. an abscess or other evidence of infection involving deep incision that is detected on gross anatomical or histopathologic exam, or imaging test.

Table 8.1 Examples of implantable device and prostheses infection definitions—cont'd

Country/ organisation	Subcategory	Overview of definition
	Organ/space SSI	Date of event occurs within 30 or 90 days after the NHSN operative procedure (where day 1 = the procedure day) according to the list in Table 2 *[of the source document]* (specific procedures are listed) AND involves any part of the body deeper than the fascial muscle layers that is opened or manipulated during the operative procedure AND patient has at least one of the following: a. purulent drainage from a drain that is placed into the organ/space (e.g. closed suction drainage system, open drain, T-tube drain, CT-guided drainage) b. organism(s) identified from fluid or tissue in the organ/space by a culture or non-culture-based microbiologic testing method which is performed for purposes of clinical diagnosis or treatment (e.g. not Active Surveillance Culture/Testing [ACT/AST]) c. an abscess or other evidence of infection involving the organ/space that is detected on gross anatomical or histopathologic exam, or imaging test evidence suggestive of infection AND meets at least one criterion for a specific organ/space infection site listed in Table 3 *[of the source document]* (specific procedures are listed).
Europe (ECDC)[9]	Superficial incisional	Infection occurs within 30 days after the operation and involves only skin and subcutaneous tissue of the incision and at least one of the following: • purulent drainage with or without laboratory confirmation, from the superficial incision • organisms isolated from an aseptically obtained culture of fluid or tissue from the superficial incision • at least one of the following signs or symptoms of infection: pain or tenderness, localised swelling, redness or heat and superficial incision is deliberately opened by surgeon, unless incision is culture-negative • diagnosis of superficial incisional SSI made by surgeon or attending physician.

Continued

Table 8.1 Examples of implantable device and prostheses infection definitions—cont'd

Country/ organisation	Subcategory	Overview of definition
	Deep incisional	Infection occurs within 30 days after the operation if no implant[†] is left in place or within 90 days if implant is in place and the infection appears to be related to the operation and infection involves deep soft tissue (e.g. fascia, muscle) of the incision and at least one of the following: • purulent drainage from the deep incision but not from the organ/space component of the surgical site • a deep incision spontaneously dehisces or is deliberately opened by a surgeon when the patient has at least one of the following signs or symptoms: fever (> 38°C), localised pain or tenderness, unless incision is culture-negative • an abscess or other evidence of infection involving the deep incision is found on direct examination, during reoperation or by histopathologic or radiologic examination • diagnosis of deep incisional SSI made by a surgeon or attending physician.
	Organ/space	Infection occurs within 30 days after the operation if no implant[†] is left in place or 90 days if implant is in place and the infection appears to be related to the operation and infection involves any part of the anatomy (e.g. organs and spaces) other than the incision that was opened or manipulated during an operation and at least one of the following: • purulent discharge from a drain that is placed through a stab wound into the organ/space • organisms isolated from an aseptically obtained culture of fluid or tissue in the organ/space • an abscess or other evidence of infection involving the organ/space that is found on direct examination, during reoperation or by histopathologic or radiologic examination • diagnosis of organ/space SSI made by a surgeon or attending physician.

*The term physician for the purpose of application of the NHSN SSI criteria may be interpreted to mean a surgeon, infectious disease physician, emergency physician, other physician on the case, or physician's designee (nurse practitioner or physician's assistant).

†The United States' National Nosocomial Infection Surveillance definition: a non-human-derived implantable foreign body (e.g. prosthetic heart valve, non-human vascular graft, mechanical heart or hip prosthesis) that is permanently placed in a patient during surgery.

Note: CDC = Centers for Disease Control. ECDC = European Centre for Disease Prevention and Control. NHSN = National Healthcare Safety Network. SSI = surgical site infection.

1. Healthcare-associated infection due to hospital-acquired complication (HAI HAC) data

Data on HAI HACs in Australia are collected by the Independent Hospital Pricing Authority (IHPA) but are not currently reported or publicly available. These data were provided upon request. The jurisdictions did not grant permission to publish the raw data but gave permission to report data by proportions. The number of HAI HACs are thus presented as a proportion. The raw data from which these proportions were calculated were provided by the IHPA.[10]

The burden of infections associated with prosthetics and implantable devices in Australian public hospitals, as identified by HAI HAC data, by state and territory for 2017–2018 and 2018–2019 is presented in Table 8.2 and Figure 8.1. Over both time periods, 77% to 80% of reported infections associated with prosthetics and implantable devices occurred in New South Wales, Victoria and Queensland (the most populous states). Proportions of infections associated with prosthetics and implantable devices (%) in the jurisdictions across the periods were generally consistent.

2. Jurisdictional HAI data

Australian jurisdictions do not undertake surveillance on prosthetic or implantable devices other than hip and knee joint replacement surgery, and these have been replicated from Chapter 2 Surgical site infection in Table 8.3.

Table 8.2 Nationwide distribution of HAI HAC associated with prosthetics and implantable devices by jurisdiction (%)

Jurisdiction	Timeframe	
	1 July 2017 – 30 June 2018	*1 July 2018 – 30 June 2019*
NSW	31.8	33.6
Vic.	19.4	23.2
Qld	26.4	22.3
SA	9.1	7.9
WA	7.4	7.6
Tas.	2.2	2.4
NT	2.0	1.4
ACT	1.6	1.6

Note: ACT = Australian Capital Territory. NSW = New South Wales. NT = Northern Territory. Qld = Queensland. SA = South Australia. Tas. = Tasmania. Vic. = Victoria. WA = Western Australia.
(Source: Compiled from IHPA data.)

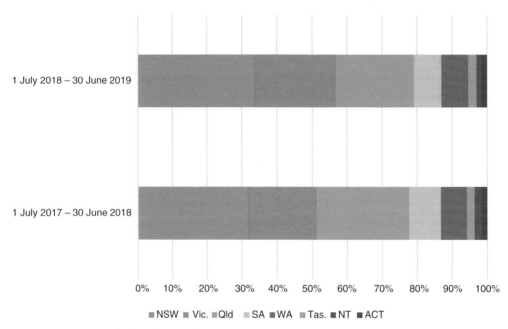

Figure 8.1 *Nationwide distribution of HAI HAC associated with prosthetics and implantable devices by jurisdiction (%)*
Note: ACT = Australian Capital Territory. NSW = New South Wales. NT = Northern Territory. Qld = Queensland. SA = South Australia. Tas. = Tasmania. Vic. = Victoria. WA = Western Australia.
(Source: Compiled from IHPA data.)

3. Peer-reviewed literature data

The final data source for infections associated with implantable devices and prostheses in Australia is the peer-reviewed literature. The findings from articles identified in the peer-reviewed literature are summarised in Table 8.4, with the definitions used detailed in Table 8.5. Only one paper reported on infections associated with prostheses and this paper considered humidity as a risk factor in prosthetic joint infection in the Australian tropics in Queensland.[13] The Australian Commission on Safety and Quality in Health Care (ACSQHC) definition of infection was used in the study.[14]

Synthesis and summary

Publicly available Australian data relating to infections associated with implantable devices and prostheses is very limited. Despite the significant morbidity and mortality reported globally in relation to these infections, the only state and territory jurisdictions publishing any data are Victoria and Western Australia and then only data relating to total joint replacement.

Table 8.3 Surgical site infection data on hip and knee joint replacement surgery

Procedure	ACT	NSW	NT	Qld	SA	Tas.	Vic.[11]	WA[12]
Hip replacement/ hip arthroplasty	–	–	–	–	–	–	2017/18 Total infections. Low risk 0.6 ($n = 354$) Higher risk 0.4 ($n = 478$) Highest risk 0.5 ($n = 189$)	2017/18 Total infections Risk all: 0.63 ($n = 315$) Risk index 0: 0.54 ($n = 2600$) Risk index 1: 0.89 ($n = 1682$) Risk index 2: 2.74 ($n = 219$) Risk index 3: 0 ($n = 17$)
Knee replacement/knee arthroplasty	–	–	–	–	–	–	2017/18 Total infections. Low risk 2.8 ($n = 1574$) Higher risk 4.6 ($n = 583$)	2017/18 Total infections Risk all: 0.8 ($n = 377$) Risk index 0: 0.43 ($n = 3708$) Risk index 1: 0.64 ($n = 2671$) Risk index 2: 1.77 ($n = 451$) Risk index 3: 10.0 ($n = 20$)
Risk index definitions	–	–	–	–	–	–	Lowest risk: undefined Low risk: undefined Higher risk: undefined Highest risk: undefined	Risk stratification is based on the CDC NHSN (United States) risk index. Risk 'All' applies to HISWA hospitals that perform fewer than 100 procedures annually and are not required to assign a risk index score. Procedure type: primary and revision.

Note: – indicates that data was not available.

Table 8.4 Data on prosthetics and implantable devices identified from literature research

Lead author	Year	Location (no. of hospitals)	Year(s) study was undertaken	Population	Type of HAI monitored	Key findings
Armit[13]	2018	Qld (1)	1999–2013	Total knee arthroplasty patients	Postoperative prosthetic joint infections	2.70%
Jarratt[15]	2013	SA (1)	2003–2011	All hospital	Medical device infection	MRO: 5 (4.9%); non-MRO: 93 (10.1%)
Phan[16]	2016	ACT (1)	2006–2010	All hospital	External ventricular drain infections	2006–2007: 9 (20.93%); 2007–2010: 13 (11.50%)

Note: ACT = Australian Capital Territory. MRO = multi-resistant organism. Qld = Queensland. SA = South Australia.

Table 8.5 HAI definitions used in the identified studies

Lead author	Year	HAI definition used
Armit[13]	2018	Deep prosthetic joint infection diagnosed using ACSQHC criteria for deep incisional/organ space infection, mirroring CDC guidelines
Jarratt[15]	2013	Defined as any localised or systemic condition resulting from an infectious agent or toxin for which no evidence was apparent on admission to the acute care setting
Phan[16]	2016	As positive microbial growth from a cerebrospinal fluid sample

The HAC data do not provide any further clarity as the devices included in the data are not defined and there are no denominator data. The peer-reviewed literature is also lacking in this area for Australia. Only one publication specifically related to prosthetics.[13] The other publications[15,16] dealt with the relationship between patient characteristics and the development of a multi-resistant HAI where infections associated with medical devices was mentioned but not further defined and a study of extra-ventricular drains which are not considered implantable devices as defined in this chapter.

At the time of writing, there is a lack of publicly available data on infections associated with implantable devices and prostheses in Australia and therefore it is difficult to quantify the burden of this category of HAI and what, if any, controls are required.

References

1. Wolford HM, Hatfield KM, Paul P, et al. The projected burden of complex surgical site infections following hip and knee arthroplasties in adults in the United States, 2020 through 2030. *Infect Control Hosp Epidemiol* 2018; **39**(10): 1189–95.

2. Rahman R, Saba S, Bazaz R, et al. Infection and readmission rate of cardiac implantable electronic device insertions: An observational single center study. *Am J Infect Control* 2016; **44**(3): 278–82.

3. National Healthcare Safety Network. Surveillance for Surgical Site Infection (SSI) Events. Atlanta: Centers for Disease Control; 2020.

4. Romero-Palacios A, Petruccelli D, Main C, et al. Screening for and decolonization of *Staphylococcus aureus* carriers before total joint replacement is associated with lower *S. aureus* prosthetic joint infection rates. *Am J Infect Control* 2019.

5. Hamilton WG, Balkam CB, Purcell RL, et al. Operating room traffic in total joint arthroplasty: Identifying patterns and training the team to keep the door shut. *Am J Infect Control* 2018; **46**(6): 633–6.

6. Edmiston CE, Jr., Chitnis AS, Lerner J, et al. Impact of patient comorbidities on surgical site infection within 90 days of primary and revision joint (hip and knee) replacement. *Am J Infect Control* 2019; **47**(10): 1225–32.

7. Ling F, Halabi S, Jones C. Comparison of air exhausts for surgical body suits (space suits) and the potential for periprosthetic joint infection. *J Hosp Infect* 2018; **99**(3): 279–83.

8. Teo BJX, Woo YL, Phua JKS, et al. Laminar flow does not affect risk of prosthetic joint infection after primary total knee replacement in Asian patients. *J Hosp Infect* 2020; **104**(3): 305–8.

9. European Centre for Disease Prevention and Control. Surveillance of surgical site infections and prevention indicators in European hospitals - HAISSI protocol. Solna: European Centre for Disease Prevention and Control; 2017.

10. Independent Hospital Pricing Authority. Healthcare-associated infections Hospital-acquired complication (HAI HAC) data. In: Independent Hospital Pricing Authority, editor. Sydney, Australia: Independent Hospital Pricing Authority; 2020.

11. Department of Health and Human Services, The University of Melbourne, The Royal Melbourne Hospital, The Peter Doherty Institute for Infection and Immunity. Healthcare-associated infection in Victoria: Surveillance report for 2016–17 and 2017–18. Melbourne, Australia, 2018.

12. Communicable Disease Control Directorate. Healthcare Infection Surveillance Western Australia: Annual Report 2017–18. Perth, Western Australia, 2018.

13. Armit D, Vickers M, Parr A, et al. Humidity a potential risk factor for prosthetic joint infection in a tropical Australian hospital. *ANZ J Surg* 2018; **88**(12): 1298–301.

14. Care ACoSaQiH. Approaches to surgical site infection surveillance: For acute care settings in Australia. Sydney: Australian Commission on Safety and Quality in Health Care; 2017.

15. Jarratt LS, Miller ER. The relationship between patient characteristics and the development of a multi-resistant healthcare-associated infection in a private South Australian hospital. *Healthc Inf* 2013; **18**(3): 94–101.

16. Phan K, Schultz K, Huang C, et al. External ventricular drain infections at the Canberra Hospital: A retrospective study. *J Clin Neurosci* 2016; **32**: 95–8.

CHAPTER 9

Gastrointestinal infection

Contents

Introduction

Although it is possible for a range of pathogens responsible for gastrointestinal infections to be transmitted within the healthcare setting, *Clostridium difficile* is the most common cause of healthcare–associated diarrhoea.[1] *C. difficile* has been responsible for outbreaks of severe disease and specific hypervirulent strains of *C. difficile* have been associated with significant morbidity and mortality.[2–4]

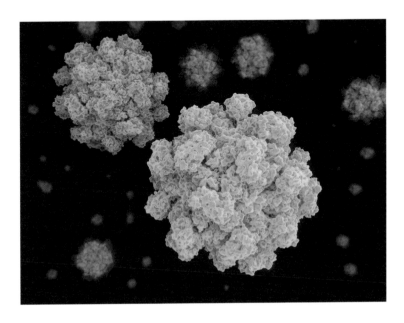

The Australian Commission on Safety and Quality in Health Care (ACSQHC) considers the rate of healthcare-associated *Clostridium difficile* infection (CDI) in a hospital to be a marker of the effectiveness of the facility's infection prevention and control program.[5] The spore-forming nature of the organism, in conjunction with the diffuse nature of diarrhoea associated with this infection, creates significant infection prevention and control challenges in relation to environmental hygiene and patient management. In the United States, around 12% of healthcare-associated infections (HAI) are related to CDI.[6] Surveillance systems have been established in the United States and Europe to monitor the epidemiology of CDI. In the United States surveillance is laboratory-based while in Europe clinical case finding is undertaken.

Given the serious sequelae associated with some strains of *C. difficile*, a range of prevention and control strategies have been implemented including:
- early identification, isolation and testing of patients with diarrhoeal disease
- enhanced environmental cleaning and disinfection
- judicious use of antimicrobials
- surveillance and case finding to identify outbreaks.[2,5,6]

This chapter presents the publicly available Australian data on CDI.

Definitions and context

The definition of gastrointestinal infections varies according to country; however, examples of gastrointestinal surveillance definitions are provided on the following pages. For further and more detailed explanations and their applications, please refer to the source document referenced.

There is no nationally agreed Australian definition for gastrointestinal infections generally; however, a definition of hospital-identified CDI was developed for the purposes of providing a standardised case definition as a basis for surveillance to monitor the epidemiology of the disease within Australia. The definition is provided in Table 9.1.

Findings

This report presents a collation and analysis of the three types of Australian data for gastrointestinal infections, including *C. difficile* infection: 1. proportions of hospital-acquired complication (HAC) data for the period 1 July 2017 to 30 June 2019; 2. publicly available state and territory jurisdiction surveillance data for the period 1 July 2016 to 30 June 2018; and 3. peer-reviewed literature data for the period 1 January 2010 to 31 August 2019. Each of these potential data sources were interrogated to gain insight into the incidence of HAI gastrointestinal infections in Australia and the findings are presented on the following pages.

Table 9.1 Examples of CDI definitions

Country/ organisation	Subcategory	Overview of definition
Australia[5]	**Hospital-identified *C. difficile* infection definition** A case of diarrhoea (i.e. an unformed stool that takes the shape of the container) that meets the following criteria: • the stool sample yields a positive result in a laboratory assay for *C. difficile* infection toxin A and/or B, or • a toxin-producing *C. difficile* organism is detected in the stool sample by culture or other means. A hospital-identified CDI case is: • a case diagnosed in a patient attending an acute care facility (i.e. it includes a positive specimen obtained from admitted patients and those attending the Emergency Department and outpatient departments). Exclusions: • cases where a known previous positive test has been obtained within the last 8 weeks (i.e. only include cases once in an 8-week period) • patients less than 2 years old. Note: An additional positive test obtained from a specimen collected from the same patient more than 8 weeks since the last positive test is regarded as a new case.	No nationally agreed or defined surveillance definition for gastrointestinal infections. The Australian Commission on Safety and Quality in Health Care (ACSQHC) has developed a definition around hospital-identified CDI.
United States CDC NHSN[7]		No nationally agreed or defined surveillance definition for gastrointestinal infections; CDI infection surveillance is laboratory-based.

Continued

Table 9.1 Examples of CDI definitions—cont'd

Country/organisation	Subcategory	Overview of definition
Europe (ECDC)[8]	**CDI surveillance definition** A case of *Clostridium difficile* infection (CDI) (previously also referred to as *C. difficile* associated diarrhoea or CDAD) must meet at least one of the following criteria: • diarrhoeal stools or toxic megacolon AND a positive laboratory assay for *C. difficile* toxin A and/or B in stools or a toxin-producing *C. difficile* organism detected in stool via culture or other means (e.g. a positive PCR result) OR • pseudomembranous colitis revealed by lower gastrointestinal endoscopy OR • colonic histopathology characteristic of *C. difficile* infection (with or without diarrhoea) on a specimen obtained during endoscopy, colectomy or autopsy.	No nationally agreed or defined surveillance definition for gastrointestinal infections generally.

1. Healthcare-associated infection due to hospital-acquired complication (HAI HAC) data

Data on HAI HACs in Australia are collected by the Independent Hospital Pricing Authority (IHPA) but are not currently reported or publicly available. These data were provided upon request. The jurisdictions did not grant permission to publish the raw data but gave permission to report data by proportions. The number of HAI HACs gastrointestinal infections are thus presented as a proportion. The raw data from which these proportions were calculated were provided by the IHPA.[9]

The burden of gastrointestinal infections in Australian public hospitals, as identified by HAI HAC data, by state and territory for 2017–2018 and 2018–2019, is presented in Table 9.2 and Figure 9.1. New South Wales, Victoria and Queensland (the most populous states) reported 77% of the gastrointestinal infections over both periods. In 2018–2019, gastrointestinal infections reported in Victoria increased by 5%, while Queensland saw a decrease by 6.5%. Proportions of gastrointestinal infections (%) in other jurisdictions over the time periods were generally consistent.

2. Jurisdictional HAI data

The second potential source of data relating to gastrointestinal infections in Australian hospitals is from data published by the Australian state and territory health departments.

Table 9.2 Nationwide distribution of HAC HAI gastrointestinal infections by jurisdiction (%)

Jurisdiction	Timeline	
	1 July 2017 – 30 June 2018	*1 July 2018 – 30 June 2019*
NSW	30.3	31.8
Vic.	25.0	30.2
Qld	21.7	15.2
SA	9.7	8.1
WA	7.5	7.5
Tas.	3.4	3.3
NT	0.5	0.8
ACT	1.9	3.2

Note: ACT = Australian Capital Territory. NSW = New South Wales. NT = Northern Territory. Qld = Queensland.
  SA = South Australia. Tas. = Tasmania. Vic. = Victoria. WA = Western Australia.
(Source: Compiled from IHPA data.)

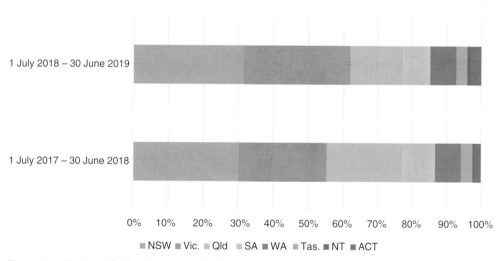

Figure 9.1 *Nationwide distribution of HAC HAI gastrointestinal infections by jurisdiction (%)*
Note: ACT = Australian Capital Territory. NSW = New South Wales. NT = Northern Territory. Qld = Queensland.
SA = South Australia. Tas. = Tasmania. Vic. = Victoria. WA = Western Australia.
(Source: Compiled from IHPA data.)

A search of each jurisdictional website was undertaken to locate any data published on gastrointestinal infections. To ensure accurate representation of the published data, each jurisdiction was contacted and asked to provide the data collected and publicly available on a range of HAI including gastrointestinal infections. The results of the searches and data provided on request are presented in Table 9.3. Some jurisdictions did not provide data.

Table 9.3 Publicly available jurisdictional hospital-identified *C. difficile* data for 2017–2018

Gastrointestinal infection	ACT	NSW	NT	Qld	SA	Tas.[10,11]	Vic.[12]	WA[13]
Clostridium difficile infection	–	–	–	–	–	2016–2017 = 5.0 cases per 10,000 patient days 2017–2018 = 5.7 cases per 10,000 patient days	2016–2017 = 2.1 cases per 10,000 OBD 2017–2018 = 1.7 cases per 10,000 OBD	2017–2018 = 5.1 cases per 10,000 OBD
						Uses ACSQHC definition[5]	Uses ACSQHC definition[5]	Uses ACSQHC definition[5]

Note: – indicates data was not provided. ACSQHC = Australian Commission on Safety and Quality in Health Care. ACT = Australian Capital Territory. NSW = New South Wales. NT = Northern Territory. OBD = occupied bed days. Qld = Queensland. SA = South Australia. Tas. = Tasmania. Vic. = Victoria. WA = Western Australia.

3. Peer-reviewed literature data

The final data source for Australian healthcare-associated CDI is the peer-reviewed literature. The findings from articles identified in the peer-reviewed literature are summarised in Table 9.4. Four articles were found that report on *C. difficile* infection incidence or prevalence. Of these, only one study reported on CDI from all states and territories except the Northern Territory, two studies reported on CDI in Victoria and one on CDI in Western Australia. There were no studies identified reporting on CDI in the Northern Territory. Infection definitions used in the studies (detailed in Table 9.5) varied and included:

- laboratory confirmation of *C. difficile* in a diarrhoeal specimen[1,14,15]
- laboratory confirmation of *C. difficile* toxin up to 60 days post hospital discharge.[2]

Due to variation between study methods, population groups and definitions comparison is not possible.

Synthesis and summary

There are a range of infections, such as norovirus and adenovirus, that occur in healthcare settings but are not included in routine surveillance. When reported in the literature, they are done so in the context of outbreaks. Although CDI is not the most common HAI, its significance in terms of morbidity and mortality and the challenges associated with environmental cleaning and disinfection means that data on CDI are more likely to be collected and published. However, such data is only

Table 9.4 Data on Clostridium difficile infections identified from literature research

Lead author	Year	Location (no. of hospitals)	Year(s) study was undertaken	Population	Type of HAI monitored	Key finding
Foster[15]	2014	WA (2)	2011–2012	All hospital	CDI	RPH: 5.2–8.1 cases/10,000 OBDs SCGH: 3.9–16.3 cases/10,000 OBDs
Hebbard[16]	2017	Vic. (2)	2013–2015	50 patients with CDI at a cancer centre	CDI	40/200 CDI cases were HA. 6.1 HA CDI episodes (95% CI: 4.7–7.7) per 10,000 OBDs
Slimings[2]	2014	ACT, Tas., Vic., NSW, Qld, SA, WA (450)	2011–2012	All hospital	CDI HA CDI: ACT, NSW, Qld, SA, Tas., Vic., WA	ACT: 5.24/10,000 patient days (95% CI: 4.61–5.95). 307 HI (hospital-identified cases incl. HA CI, non-HA CDI, CA CDI) per 10,000 patient days. NSW: N/A; 4674 HI per 10,000 patient days Qld: N/A; 1250 HI per 10,000 patient days SA: 2.53/10,000 patient days (95% CI: 2.33–2.75); 1216 HI per 10,000 patient days Tas.: 3.36/10,000 patient days (95% CI: 2.91–3.85); 357 HI per 10,000 patient days Vic.: 2.83/10,000 patient days (95% CI: 2.72–2.94); 3411 HI per 10,000 patient days WA: 3.21/10,000 patient days (95% CI: 3.00–3.44); 1468 HI per 10,000 patient days NT: 2.95/10,000 patient days (95% CI: 2.86–3.04); 4446 HI per 10,000 patient days.
Worth[1]	2016	Vic. (136)	2010–2014	All hospital	CDI	2.49/10,000 OBDs; 4826 CDI events

Note: ACT = Australian Capital Territory. HA = healthcare-associated. HI = hospital-identified. NT= Northern Territory. OBDs = occupied bed days. Qld = Queensland. RPH = Royal Perth Hospital. SA = South Australia. SCGH = Sir Charles Gairdner Hospital. Tas. = Tasmania. Vic. = Victoria. WA = Western Australia. (*Source: Compiled from IHPA data.*)

Table 9.5 HAI definitions used in the identified studies

Lead author	Year	HAI definition used
Foster[15]	2014	Patients were classified as having 'laboratory-confirmed CDI' if they experienced the passage of three or more unformed or loose stools conforming to the shape of a container (diarrhoea) within a 24-hour period and had a *C. difficile*-positive laboratory test result
Hebbard[16]	2017	Consistent with national surveillance methods, categories included healthcare facility (HCF) associated; healthcare facility onset (symptom onset more than 48 hours after admission to HCF), HCF-associated, community-onset (symptom onset within community or within 48 hours of admission to HCF, providing onset was within 4 weeks of last discharge from HCF); community associated (symptom onset in community or within 48 hours of admission to HCF, provided last admission to HCF was more than 12 weeks prior); indeterminate if onset didn't fulfil these criteria
Slimings[2]	2014	National definition of CDI; hospital-identified CDI defined as CDI diagnosed in a patient attending any area of an acute public hospital; CDI case was defined as a patient having diarrhoea, and the stool sample yielded a positive result in a laboratory assay for *C. difficile* toxin A and/or B, or a toxin-producing strain of *C. difficile* was detected in the stool sample by culture or PCR
Worth[1]	2016	All cases of laboratory-confirmed CDI were included in the surveillance; a positive result for *C. difficile* toxin A or B or the presence of a toxin-producing *C. difficile* organism in a diarrhoeal specimen was required for diagnosis of CDI; healthcare-associated, HCF onset defined as > 48 hours after admission; healthcare-associated, community-onset defined as onset within 48 hours of HCF admission and within 4 weeks of discharge from a HCF

Note: CDI = *Clostridium difficile* infection. HAI = healthcare-associated infection. HCF = healthcare facility. PCR = polymerase chain reaction.

published by three Australian states, making it difficult to establish and track the epidemiology of this infection over time. The data that are published by Victoria and Western Australia provide hospital-identified cases of CDI which, by definition, could include community-acquired cases of disease. The same approach is taken by Tasmania; however, the data are further refined to identify the proportion of cases that are healthcare-associated with healthcare facility onset.

Results derived from HAC data are based on the interpretation of clinical records. They remain unvalidated and the gastrointestinal infections included are not defined. Furthermore, those data as they have been provided represent only the proportion of the gastrointestinal infections contributed by each jurisdiction to the whole and the organism(s) causing the infection is not identified.

The peer-reviewed literature reporting on the Australian experience with CDI varied in focus with two papers reporting on the epidemiology of CDI in Victoria and Western Australia respectively, while a third paper reported on the risk factors for CDI infection and outcomes in a matched case-control cohort of cancer patients. The final paper presented the results of a systematic review and meta-analysis of the associations between antibiotic classes and hospital-acquired CDI.

At the time of writing, there is a paucity of publicly available data on healthcare-associated CDI in Australia and therefore the epidemiology of the disease is difficult to determine. This is surprising, in light of the consequences of severe disease, and the fact that *C. difficile* is the most common cause of healthcare-associated diarrhoea.

References

1. Worth LJ, Spelman T, Bull AL, et al. Epidemiology of *Clostridium difficile* infections in Australia: enhanced surveillance to evaluate time trends and severity of illness in Victoria, 2010–2014. *J Hosp Infect* 2016; **93**(3): 280–5.
2. Slimings C, Riley TV. Antibiotics and hospital-acquired *Clostridium difficile* infection: update of systematic review and meta-analysis. *J Antimicrob Chemother* 2014; **69**(4): 881–91.
3. Herbert R, Hatcher J, Jauneikaite E, et al. Two-year analysis of *Clostridium difficile* ribotypes associated with increased severity. *J Hosp Infect* 2019; **103**(4): 388–94.
4. Honda H, Kato H, Olsen MA, et al. Risk factors for *Clostridioides difficile* infection in hospitalized patients and associated mortality in Japan: a multi-centre prospective cohort study. *J Hosp Infect* 2020; **104**(3): 350–7.
5. Australian Commission on Safety and Quality in Health Care. CDI Implementation Guide for Surveillance of *Clostridium difficile* infection. Sydney: Australian Commission on Safety and Quality in Health Care; 2013.
6. Barker AK, Zellmer C, Tischendorf J, et al. On the hands of patients with *Clostridium difficile*: A study of spore prevalence and the effect of hand hygiene on *C. difficile* removal. *Am J Infect Control* 2017; **45**(10): 1154–6.
7. National Healthcare Safety Network. Short Summary: Testing for *C. difficile* and Standardized Infection Ratios, National Healthcare Safety Network, 2019: Centers for Disease Control and Prevention, 2019.
8. European Centre for Disease Prevention and Control. European Surveillance of *Clostridium difficile* infections. Surveillance protocol version 2.2. Solan: European Centre for Disease Prevention and Control 2015.
9. Independent Hospital Pricing Authority. Healthcare-associated infections Hospital-acquired complication (HAI HAC) data. In: Independent Hospital Pricing Authority, editor. Sydney, Australia: Independent Hospital Pricing Authority; 2020.
10. Wilson F, Anderson T, Wells A. Tasmanian Acute Public Hospitals Healthcare Associated Infection Report No 34—Annual Report 2016–17. In: Services DoHaH, editor. Hobart: Department of Health and Human Services, Tasmania; 2017. p. 47.
11. Wilson F, Anderson T, Wells A. Tasmanian Acute Public Hospitals Healthcare Associated Infection Report No 38—Annual Report 2017–18. In: Services DoHaH, editor. Hobart: Department of Health and Human Services, Tasmania; 2018. p. 43.
12. Department of Health and Human Services, The University of Melbourne, The Royal Melbourne Hospital, The Peter Doherty Institute for Infection and Immunity. Healthcare-associated infection in Victoria: Surveillance report for 2016–17 and 2017–18. Melbourne, Australia, 2018.
13. Communicable Disease Control Directorate. Healthcare Infection Surveillance Western Australia: Annual Report 2017–18. Perth, Western Australia, 2018.

14. Australian Commission on Safety and Quality in Health Care. Hospital-acquired Complications (HACs) List. Version 3.0 ed. Sydney: Australian Commission on Safety and Quality in Health Care; 2019.

15. Foster NF, Collins DA, Ditchburn SL, et al. Epidemiology of *Clostridium difficile* infection in two tertiary-care hospitals in Perth, Western Australia: a cross-sectional study. *New Microbes New Infect* 2014; **2**(3): 64–71.

16. Hebbard AIT, Slavin MA, Reed C, et al. Risks factors and outcomes of *Clostridium difficile* infection in patients with cancer: a matched case-control study. *Support Care Cancer* 2017; **25**(6): 1923–30.

CHAPTER 10

Appendix

Contents

Introduction

The purpose of this monograph is to collate the available data regarding the epidemiology of healthcare–associated infection (HAI) in Australia. The following methods were adopted for data collection.

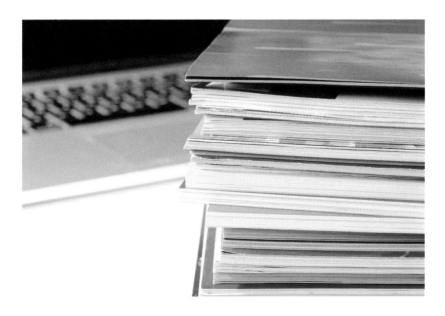

Hospital-acquired complication data

The Australian Commission on Safety and Health Care (ACSQHC) describes a hospital-acquired complication (HAC) as a complication associated with the provision of healthcare where the application of clinical risk-mitigation strategies may reduce (but not necessarily eliminate) the risk of the complication.[1] There are 16 types of HACs, one of which is HAI related.

HAC data are based on clinical coding information. Clinical coders review the patient record and look for information in the record to codify all the elements of admitted patient care provided, based on a system of medical diagnosis codes.

In Australia, all HAC-related code(s) are derived from the Australian Coding Standards (ACS), *International Statistical Classification of Diseases and Related Health Problems* (10th revision), Australian Modification (ICD-10-AM) and Australian Classification of Health Interventions (ACHI). This classification system is referred to as *ICD-10-AM/ACHI/ACS*. Starting 1 July 2019, the *ICD-10-AM/ACHI/ACS* Eleventh Edition was implemented.[2]

Collection and monitoring of HAC data is performed by all Australian states and territories. HAC data from all Australian adult and paediatric public hospitals are stored on the National Benchmarking Portal,[3] a secure online application hosted by the Independent Hospital Pricing Authority (IHPA). This data is not publicly available and access to the data is dependent upon approval from all the jurisdictions. All requests for data access and release for the purposes of research must go through IHPA. In addition to IHPA, the Australian Institute of Health and Welfare (AIHW) also hosts public hospital data collections on its online metadata registry, METeOR.[4]

In this monograph, the *ICD-10-AM/ACHI/ACS* Tenth Edition[5] and HACs specification V2.0 July 2019[6] were used for coding all HAI HAC data. This edition was implemented between 1 July 2017 and 30 June 2019. In accordance with this 10th edition, the ACSQHC listed the following eight diagnoses as subcategories of HAIs:

1. urinary tract infection
2. surgical site infection
3. pneumonia
4. bloodstream infection
5. central line and peripheral line associated bloodstream infection
6. multi-resistant organism
7. infection associated with prosthetics/implantable devices
8. gastrointestinal infection.

In September 2019, the authors approached AIHW and IHPA with requests to access all HAC HAI data from all Australian public and private hospitals for the two periods: 1 July 2017 to 30 June 2018 and 1 July 2018 to 30 June 2019. Data requested did not contain accompanying denominator data and only contains episode counts with a HAC. Australian Refined Diagnosis Related Groups (AR-DRGs) classification were not provided. The raw data from which these proportions were calculated were provided by IHPA upon request but are not publicly available. Permission was granted to publish only the epidemiology of the eight HAI HACs as a proportion. The proportions that are presented in this title are expressed to one decimal point, and as such the totals for each jurisdiction may not equal 100% exactly due to rounding after the decimal point.

Jurisdictional HAI data

Broad variation exists in the type of jurisdictional HAI data that are collated and publicly available. Where it is available, the mode in which it is disseminated is also inconsistent across jurisdictions. A number of steps were taken to identify jurisdictional HAI data. Initially, all jurisdictional infection prevention health-related websites were searched. This resulted in variable success. Where it did exist, differences in infection type, denominators and timeframes limited its usefulness.

In November 2019 at the Australasian College for Infection Prevention and Control conference in Perth, a representative from each jurisdiction presented data from their jurisdictional surveillance activities. Following the conference, each jurisdictional presenter was contacted via email and a request was made to respond to the following questions.

1. Could you please provide a summary of the structure and function of the HAI surveillance program for your jurisdiction? A copy of your presentation from the ACIPC 2019 International Conference would more than suffice for this purpose.
2. What HAI data are collected that *are* publicly available?
3. What HAI data are collected that *are not* publicly available?
4. How, and where, can the publicly available HAI data be accessed?
5. Who collects HAI data in your jurisdiction?
6. How are HAI data transferred to you?
7. How are HAI data validated, and by whom?
8. How, where and how frequently are HAI data reported?

Publicly available data was defined as being published on jurisdictional websites or in written reports, or was otherwise available, for access by the general public without the need for special approval.

Jurisdictions that had not responded within 6 weeks were followed up with a reminder email, and then again after another 4 weeks. Not all jurisdictions were able to respond in this timeframe. When jurisdictions responded with data or references to available data, attempts were made to extract data as per the eight HAC categories listed above for the years 2017 and 2018 and any additional data after that period.

Peer-reviewed literature data

To identify peer-reviewed data on HAI incidence and prevalence in Australian hospitals, the electronic databases MEDLINE (PubMed) and the Cumulative Index to Nursing and Allied Health Literature (CINAHL) were used to undertake a systematic search for relevant articles published between 1 January 2010 and 31 August 2019. This timeframe was selected in order to provide a picture of current research and to account for the fact that, during the 2000s, a number of state and national initiatives were undertaken to reduce the rate of HAIs, including the National Hand Hygiene Initiative, development of National Health and Medical Research Council (NHMRC) guidelines, revision of hospital accreditation standards, surveillance initiatives and public reporting of some infection data. The reference lists of eligible articles that related to these initiatives were reviewed to identify potential additional articles.

Articles from MEDLINE and CINAHL were identified using the search terms 'surveillance', 'incidence', 'prevalence', 'frequency', 'rates or statistics' and 'performance indicators', in combination with 'nosocomial infection', 'hospital-acquired infection', 'associated infection', 'cross-infection' and 'infection'. To limit the search to articles relating to Australian hospitals, the search term 'hospital' was used in combination with 'Australia', 'Australian', 'Queensland', 'New South Wales', 'Australian Capital Territory', 'Victoria', 'Tasmania', 'South Australia', 'Western Australia' and 'Northern Territory'. These terms were applied using an all-text search. Searches using MEDLINE additionally used the Medical Subject Heading (MeSH) terms 'epidemiology', 'cross-infection' and 'disease transmission, infectious'.

Inclusion criteria

Articles that reported rates of HAI in cohort studies, case-control studies, cross-sectional studies, randomised controlled trials or case reports were considered eligible. To be eligible, data collection for the study needed to have occurred after 1 January 2010, and to have taken place in Australian hospitals. If a study was international or multi-centre, data from Australian hospitals were included if reported at this level. Where Australia-specific data were not available in such studies, the paper was excluded. Given the difficulties associated with defining colonisation versus infection, incidence or prevalence of multi-resistant organisms was not specifically searched for.

Exclusion criteria

All grey literature, conference abstracts, papers written in languages other than English, reviews, editorials, commentaries and policy statements were excluded. Research that involved an intervention was also excluded.

Definitions

For this report, the definition of an HAI used in the articles must have referenced a recognised standard such as a definition agreed upon and/or published by a professional association or government agency, a definition widely used in the published literature or an ICD-10 code that constitutes an HAI. Any disputes about whether an article had used an appropriate definition were resolved via discussion between the authors.

Titles and abstracts of the articles identified using MEDLINE and CINAHL were evaluated by one reviewer for relevance to the aims of the book. Articles that were then deemed irrelevant were excluded. The abstracts of a random selection (10%) of articles were independently reviewed by another reviewer to identify any discrepancies; none were identified. Of the remaining articles, a full-text review was undertaken to determine eligibility. Where there was uncertainty as to whether an article should be included, two researchers independently reviewed the articles. If there was disagreement, a third reviewer made the final assessment.

Data collection process

A data extraction form was developed from the included papers. All data items extracted were cross-checked for accuracy. No attempt was made to contact the authors of papers that had missing data or unclear information.

Risk of bias

No risk of bias assessment was undertaken.

Diagram for study selection

Figure 10.1 illustrates the process for summarising the article identified in the review of the peer-reviewed literature.

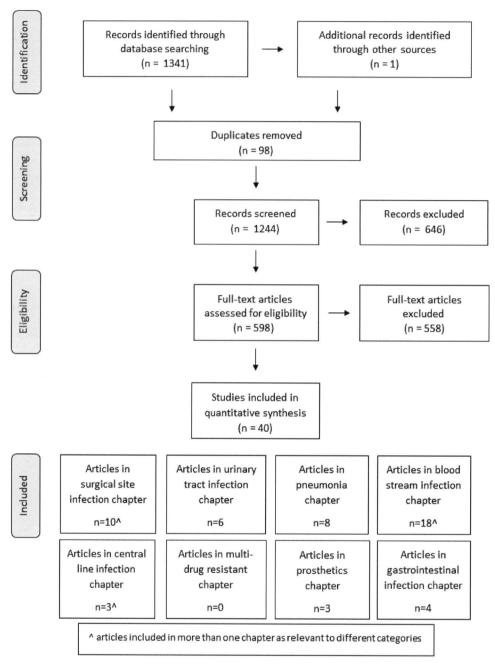

Figure 10.1 *PRISMA flow diagram for study selection* *(Source: http://www.prisma-statement.org/ PRISMAStatement/FlowDiagram.)*

References

1. Australian Commission on Safety and Quality in Health Care. Hospital-Acquired Complications Information Kit. Sydney: Australian Commission on Safety and Quality in Health Care 2018.
2. Independent Hospital Pricing Authority. ICD-10-AM/ACHI/ACS current edition 2020 (Available from: https://www.ihpa.gov.au/what-we-do/icd-10-am-achi-acs-current-edition accessed 21 April 2020).
3. Independent Hospital Pricing Authority. National Benchmarking Portal 2020 (Available from: https://www.ihpa.gov.au/what-we-do/data-collection/national-benchmarking-portal accessed 21 April 2020).
4. Australian Institute of Health and Welfare. METeOR (Metadata Online Registry) Canberra 2020 (available from: https://meteor.aihw.gov.au/content/index.phtml/itemId/181162 accessed 21 April 2020).
5. Independent Hospital Pricing Authority. ICD-10-AM/ACHI/ACS previous editions 2020 (available from: https://www.ihpa.gov.au/what-we-do/icd-10-am-achi-acs-previous-editions accessed 21 April 2020).
6. Australian Commission on Safety and Quality in Health Care. Hospital-acquired complications specifications V2.0—July 2019, 2019.